Reflection of a Survivor

Reflection of a Survivor

My Personal Journey through Breast Cancer

Karen Maneri

Copyright © 2008 by Karen Maneri.

Library of Congress Control Number:		2008903085
ISBN:	Hardcover	978-1-4363-3365-8
	Softcover	978-1-4363-3364-1

This book was printed in the United States of America.

Photographer: Micci DeBonis
(Front book cover photo and Back Author photo)
Hudson Valley Photo, Fishkill, New York 12524
HVPS1@optonline.net

Graphic Design by: Kirsten Heincke
(Design on front and back cover)
KH Creative, Inc.
Beacon, New York 12508-3806
brown_bag@verizon.net

To order additional copies of this book, contact:
Xlibris Corporation
1-888-795-4274
www.Xlibris.com
Orders@Xlibris.com
48931

Contents

Chapter Eighteen

Chapter Nineteen

Chapter Twenty

Acknowledgements

Introduction

Five years ago while enjoying a life filled with the joys and struggles many wives and working mothers of 2 year olds are faced with daily, a moment came when I knew something was not right within my own body.

At 33 I was diagnosed with breast cancer. Within minutes the realities of life I had lived for so long were about to take a sharp turn into the unknown as I began my battle with a life threatening illness that took me on a journey of a lifetime . . .

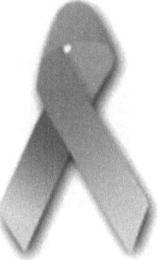

As sad as I was to loose my grandmother (Catherine Dross) and my aunt (Kathy Ritch) just weeks before my diagnosis, I whole heartily believe it was their constant presence that helped sustain my faith along the way.

Thanks for being there when I needed you most. I will forever Love You!

Foreward

In August of 1996 I was just starting my career as a stylist in a local salon. My boss was out sick and the receptionist asked if I could stay late to cut and color one of his clients. "Karen" was going on vacation the next day and was desperate to have her hair done for her trip. Apprehensively I agreed and immediately went into a state of panic when she sat in my chair and asked me to "get rid" of her long brown locks, she wanted me to make her a "blonde"!

Karen was newly single and was reinventing her life . . . starting with her trip to Florida the next day.

We spent the next 2 hours transforming her "exterior" to reflect the amazing state of growth of her "inner self". Karen left that day "loving" her new look, excited to "start over" and I went home "loving" this impressive young woman, I felt honored to have met that day.

At the young age of 26 Karen's spirit & ambition was inspiring to say the least. For the last 13 years we have redesigned Karen's hair in dozen of styles that have been as diverse as her ever evolving self. For over a decade we've grown up together sharing stories of dating disasters, finding "Mr. Right", the challenges of pursuing our careers, the excitement of buying our first homes, the joys and fears that come with pregnancies, motherhood and battling the "baby bulge". In all that time we never expected that in our early 30's one of us having BREAST CANCER would be added to the long list of life experiences we'd shared.

Karen called on a busy Saturday to let me know she had not been in for quite some time as she had been busy with a friends wedding and she wouldn't need her hair done anytime soon as she was starting chemotherapy because she had BREAST CANCER! I was speechless, frozen by fear, disbelief and confusion. My young healthy beautiful client now friend was speaking clearly in English on the other end of the phone. I could not comprehend what she was telling me . . . "MY KAREN" HAD BREAST CANCER?

So we spent the last few years sharing her journey into the unknown as we had shared so many of the other events in our life.

When Karen called a few months back, excited that the book she was writing was almost finished she asked if I would read it and give her some feedback. She was trying to design the cover and wanted a "readers" perspective of her writings. I asked her what she wanted the cover to express so I could keep that in mind while reading her story. She responded that she wanted people to know just by looking at the cover before they even read the book that surviving this devastating disease made her who she is today. Again I was silent . . . My response was simple, Breast Cancer in no way created who you are today. It was merely a flood light that illuminated the magnificence of who you have always been. It brought to the surface the essence of who "Karen" truly is made up of, strengths and weakness just as we all are. With everything you have learned through your journey with breast cancer the greatest gift I feel it has given you is the ability to see clearly what I have known all along. You are one of the most magnificent women I have ever met and this book celebrates the woman and spirit you have always been. You are every ones inspiration you will inspire other young women, mothers, sisters, friends, and even strangers who read your journey. Thank you Karen for inspiring me, I love you!

Jennifer Paden

Chapter One

"Why Me—Why Now"

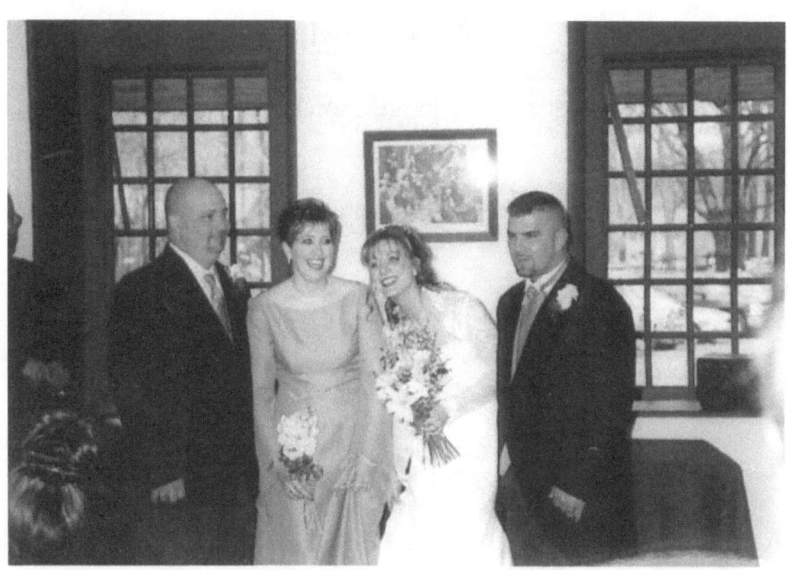

Gary (Best Man), Karen (Maid of Honor), Sandy (Bride), and Dave (Groom)

It was a warm, calm, quiet Friday evening, in May of 2003. My husband and I were lying in bed, and my two year old son was sound asleep in his room. Gary and I were watching a movie like we always do every weekend, laughing and talking. I gently ran my hand over the inner part of my right breast, and what I felt startled me. I didn't say anything to my husband at first I just kept touching the lump to see if it would go away. Then I started feeling the left side to see if maybe there was something on that side of my breast, hoping there was because then I would have felt much better. To my surprise the lump was not on the left side, I then said to my husband, "Feel this" I knew he was probably thinking to himself, "what now." I have always been obsessive with my body, and always thinking something was wrong with me when really nothing ever was. However, this time I had the most overwhelming feeling and I could not stop touching the lump in my breast. When Gary did not say anything I knew what he was thinking. He said, "Maybe you should call the doctor." Anyone who knows Gary knows that is not something he would say. "He does not even like doctors."

For the rest of the night we both were pretty silent, not saying another word. Our minds were wandering, and thinking of what it could be. Neither one of us wanted to talk about it, so we tried to pretend it was nothing. We didn't really want to accept what it may be.

What Now!

"This was one of the longest weekends of my life."

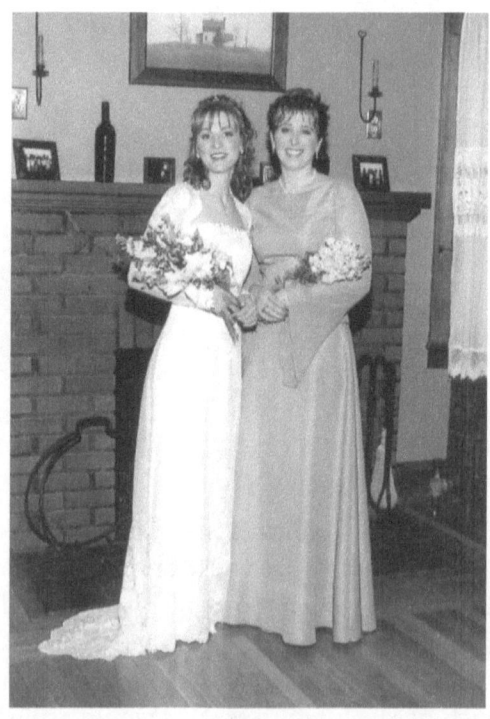

Sandy and Karen April 4, 2003

Monday came along, and I jumped out of bed, got ready for work and headed out early so I could call the doctor's office. I dropped Owen off to my mother-in-law who always watched him when I went to work. I worked three days during the week and both weekend days. I loved my job at first. I worked with the most remarkable women. I worked for a New York News paper. We handled all of the financial accounts of the customers, mass mailing of the paper, and customer service. When I arrived at work I started my day and tried to forget about the lump in my breast, but I just couldn't keep my hand off of it, I was drawn to it like a magnet. I even circled it and had all the girls at work feel it to see if they could feel what I was feeling. It made me feel better knowing that I wasn't the only person who could feel this unwelcoming lump in my breast. I began thinking "maybe it really was nothing."

When I called my gynecologist office for an appointment, the receptionist said that I could not be seen for a week. That did not sit well with me. Dr. P., (this is what I will call him) is my gynecologist, so I asked the receptionist to get him a message, call me ASAP, it was an emergency. A few hours went by and I still had not heard from the doctor. Usually when I call, he calls me right back, so I knew he probably had not received my message. I called again and demanded for the receptionist to put Dr. P., on the phone. Luckily my best friend Dawn was in the office with him; she had an exam that morning. (She had already told him what was going on), since on Saturday morning, she felt the lump too. It was making me crazy I needed as many people to feel as possible, that way I knew it wasn't just in my head. She also said I better have that looked at. Dr. P. took my call and told me to come in immediately.

I had already told my supervisor that I might have to leave for a little while for an appointment and she was okay with that. Even if she wasn't okay with me leaving I was going to leave anyway.

His Face Showed All

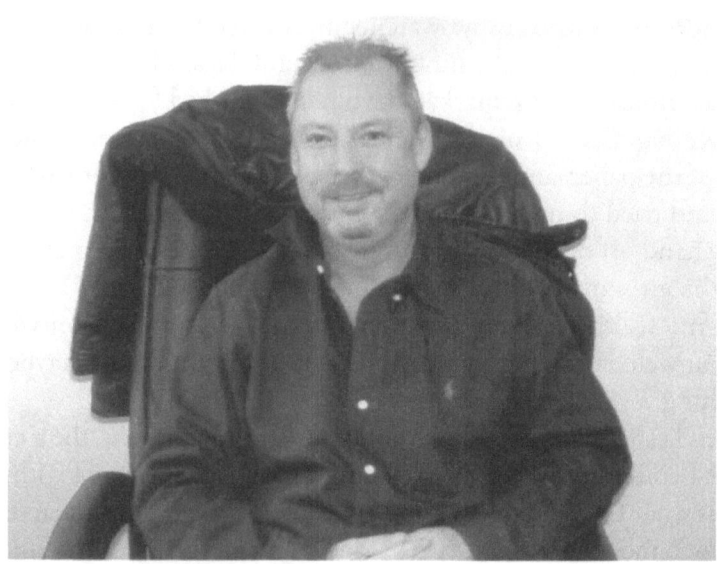

Dr. P

When I finally arrived at the doctor's office, they brought me in right away. The nurse asked me to undress from the waist up, gown open in the front. My heart was pounding, and I was sweating like crazy, the room was cold. Sitting on the table waiting in this horrible paper gown, it felt as if it was taking forever for the doctor to come in. Finally in walked Dr. P., happy as always to see me. He did the routine breast exam; I knew right away he did not really feel what I was talking about. He felt around and said, I don't think it's anything to really worry about, but, to be safe I want you to have a mammogram, ultrasound, and see a breast surgeon. I want to take all necessary precautions.

"Get dressed and meet me in my office."

As I was putting on my bra and shirt, I knew he did not feel what I felt! I started to feel for it again to make sure it was still there. I thought maybe it disappeared. But, I found it. It was in a very odd part of my breast. That's why it was so hard for the doctor to feel. I could feel it better when I was standing. When I walked into his office I closed the door, I lifted up my shirt and said please feel here. Well when he touched it, my heart sank because his face showed all. He tried hard not to show fear, but it showed. He said okay I feel it now, but it still may not be anything, but he wanted the tests done ASAP.

I believe in my heart that he knew without even having the results that I had breast cancer!

It felt like a marble in my breast, it didn't hurt or move, I wasn't feeling sick I figured maybe he's right, it probably is nothing. I went back to work and made a phone call to the Imaging center in town, the receptionist made my appointment for Wednesday, May 7. I was very happy that it was soon because the waiting was making me insane. I couldn't sleep or eat, until these tests were done.

Chapter Two

All Alone

The morning of my mammogram and ultra sound my mother wanted to know if I needed her to go with me I told her not to worry, to go to work and I would call when my appointment was over. I went by myself and sat there in the waiting room, looking around at all of the women having their mammograms and wondering if anyone else was there for the same reason. I was sure they were looking at me and wondering why I was there. I was the youngest one in the room. I dressed in the cloth gown and waited my turn. When the nurse came out to get me I was scared, but just wanted to get it over with. Just the thought of my boob being flattened in that machine was terrifying.

After my mammogram, I went into another room for my ultra sound. While having the ultra sound the tech could see the lump in my breast, much better than on the mammogram. She took quite a few measurements and pictures, and then asked me to get dressed and have a seat in the waiting room. As I was sitting there I knew that something was wrong. The radiologist came out and asked me to go with him and the nurse into a private room. "I began to panic." I said to myself this is bad! We went over the results; and he told me I had a palpable mass measuring about 1.5cm in diameter with shaggy outer margins. The ultrasound showed it to be solid so it required biopsy. He handed me the films and wished me good luck, adding if I had any concerns to please feel free to call. He told me he will send this report over to Dr. P., immediately.

I was stunned and confused, not knowing what to do. I could not believe that this was actually happening to me, how did this happen, why me?

So I got into my car and started to cry. I was by myself and in disbelief that this was really happening.

"I wanted to call Gary, but I knew he was working, I didn't want to upset him."

I was so upset I could barely drive. I am surprised I did not cause an accident. I couldn't even see straight, so I stopped at a friend's house, I needed to calm down and regroup myself. I knocked on the door, her husband answered; I just broke down crying hysterically. Nothing coming out of my mouth was making since. Christina came out from the other room and asked me, "what was wrong" I couldn't stop crying, "I was already thinking the worst, I had that gut feeling I couldn't get rid of."

I started to explain what had happened at my appointment. Joe, Christina, and I sat and talked for a while about my results. They told me not to expect the worst. They told me that everything would be alright, to try to keep my chin up and be positive.

Once I was calm enough to drive, I thanked them for listening. I told them I would call when I arrived at home, this way they knew I made it home safe. I worked with Christina and we became very good friend. She is an incredible person inside and out. We have a very close friendship, the minute I met her I knew we had a special connection.

Chapter Three

Appointment Time

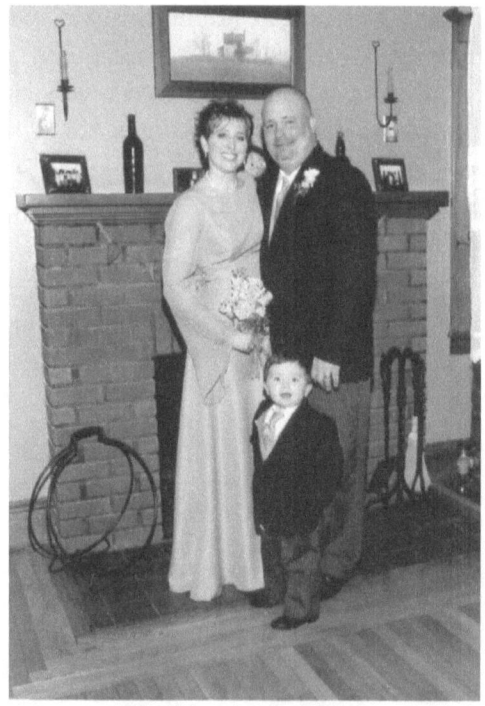

Gary, Karen and Owen

My friend Sandy is a nurse, she knew a lot of doctors to call she was on her honeymoon. Sandy and Dave were married on April 4, 2003. They left for their honeymoon April 30, and would not return until May 11.

I was her maid of honor, Gary was the best man, and Owen was the ring barer.

I couldn't call her cell phone and upset her. She was on a cruise, and I didn't want to worry her while she was so far away. Plus we really didn't know what it was, it still could be nothing. I could not wait until she came home.

Meanwhile, unbeknownst to me, Sandy was having anxiety about getting home and didn't know why. As soon as she arrived at the Boston Port she called me. The phone rang and I saw that it was her, I started to cry, I began telling her about all the tests I had already had, that I had a lump and I needed a biopsy. Then I told her I made my appointment with a local surgeon so I could have him look at the films and guide me in the next direction.

In the meantime, while this was all going on, my aunt was in the hospital dying from liver disease. She was like a mother to me, it was very hard accepting the fact that she was dying. My aunt and I had a mother-daughter bond, she had two boys so I was the daughter she never had. Part of me was glad she was not able to understand what was happening to me, it would have destroyed her. It was very difficult looking at her so sick. Seeing my two cousins so upset, they knew that she was dying and there was nothing they could do to help. Cory, her oldest son is very mature for his age; Derek is the younger of the two. They needed my mother to help them get through. Looking at both of them watching them wait for their mother to die, was heart breaking. Thinking to myself, "this could be me." I didn't want my husband and son to watch me die. I prayed that this lump would turn out to be nothing to worry about. I could not even tell my cousins that it was possible that I was sick too. They needed me they didn't need to hear that I may die too. It was way too much to handle.

So much bad news in just two weeks, my emotions were all over the place.

When Sandy came home, it was a big relief; she came directly from the Boston Port right off the ship to see me with her luggage still in the car.

She told me that she cried all the way home "her husband kept saying you do not even know if it is cancer," so why are you so upset? Stop crying?

She made arrangements to go with me to my appointment to the local surgeon the appointment was scheduled for May 12th. Gary wanted to be with us, but he had to work. It was the busiest time of the year for his job. This was no time for him to be taking time off. Plus he had no clue what any of this meant. He preferred for Sandy to be with me.

I remember we were sitting in the room looking at some pictures of what cancer looked like in someone's breast. I kept thinking, "I hope that's not me."

The surgeon came in and said, "Let me bring the films to MY radiologist and see what he thinks; I will be right back." When he returned, he said his radiologist did not think it was anything, that I was too young for breast cancer, "it's probably benign."

Sandy and I were not very happy with the doctors laid back attitude; he seemed very care free.

Chapter Four

Biopsy Day
"The Moment of Truth"

Doctor D., arranged for a biopsy for May 16 at a local hospital in Dutchess County, Friday was becoming an unlucky day for me. The biopsy was called an ultrasound guided core biopsy. A long needle is stuck into the breast, guided by an ultrasound it removes multiple pieces of the lesion, the specimen is sent out for biopsy. The tech took four samples, and then inserted a small metal clip into the breast to mark the area of the tumor so if the biopsy proves cancerous the surgeon would know exactly where it was. Even though I had been injected with Novocain in the right breast around the area of the lump the pressure and pain was awful and the whole experience was frightening. They didn't even allow anyone to be with me in the room, so it made me more nervous, "I felt so alone." I must say though the ultra sound tech and his nurse were really wonderful and caring. They explained everything that was going on, he and the nurse asked me if I had any questions, and told me what to expect in the next few days. The tech told me that the results would be back by Monday or Tuesday, to follow up with the doctor.

Three days before my biopsy my aunt passed away from cirrhosis of the liver May 13, 2003. My whole family was devastated the thought of two young boys with no mother, she was too young to die. How will these boys live without a mother? I knew my mother was thinking about me also. It was so hard to mourn the death of my aunt when I was not quite sure about my own prognosis.

After the biopsy, I went home to wait and recover. I felt like all I did the past few weeks is wait to find out, the outcome, of the rest of my life.

Monday rolled around, and I had not heard anything from the doctor. Every time the phone rang my heart just sank, "I was emotionally a mess".

Some doctors have no compassion for their patients, especially when they take their time getting important test results to you. This doctor was one who didn't seem to care.

Everyone kept telling me, the old saying is, "No news is good news." I was tired of people saying things like that. When you are waiting for the doctor to tell you if you are going to live or die, you don't want to hear what the "old saying is." I was very anxious and knew deep in my gut that this was going to be bad; I was preparing for the worst.

I just wanted to call to find out, but my husband wanted to wait one more day, and if we still hadn't heard from the doctor we would call. I went to work on Tuesday and started my day. I am not a very patient person, so when the doctors' office opened at 9:00am I started to call, and of course, the nurse was not in until 11:00am. More waiting, do they not think I have waited long enough?

I decided to take an early lunch to go home to make the call. On my way home, I called Sandy (from my cell phone) to let her know that I was coming home for lunch, to call for my biopsy results.

Something made me ask her a question. She sounded different on the phone, I asked her "are you pregnant", I have no idea why I asked that question, but something made me ask, she said, "How do you know?" I said "I just do."

When I got home, I called the doctor who ordered the biopsy. The nurse answered the phone; I told her I was waiting for my biopsy results, so I gave her my name. She said, "Let me get your paper work." She came back to the phone and said in a soft voice, "Karen you have cancer"!

I asked her to repeat what she just said; I thought I was hearing things, she said again, "you have breast cancer!"

I asked her, "Am I going to die?" It was quiet on the other end of the phone. She was not sure how to respond to that question. Does anyone know what to say to that! I asked if I could come in and see the doctor and she told me that he was out of the office and would not return for three days. I explained to her that I felt I had waited long enough, that I have a two year old son, a husband and family who need me.

I hung up the phone and started to cry. Whom do I call first? What do I do now? I called Sandy who was waiting for my call, and when she picked up the phone, I told her, "I had cancer and I was going to die," she did not say anything. I remember saying again, "I am going to die." I heard her say, I will be right there.

Chapter Five

Am I Going To Die?

I was waiting to call my husband and family. I did not know how to tell them that I had breast cancer.

The love of my life, who just four years earlier lost his father to cancer, my mother who two weeks earlier lost her sister to liver disease, and my father who lost his mother on Easter Sunday (my grandmother,) from a blood clot to the brain. Now they may lose a wife, a daughter and Owen would lose his mother. It just broke my heart to have to tell them this terrifying news. The anxiety was intense, I was sick to my stomach, I had a headache, and I felt like I could not breathe.

Waiting for Sandy to arrive seemed like an eternity. When she walked through the door we both were crying and hugging each another.

Pregnancy and Cancer!!

"What are the odds of two positive results in one day?"

The first thing I thought of was, when a child is born, another dies, "I thought it would be me." We stepped back from one another, wiped away the tears and said, "We have work to do." I called Gary who was working with Sandy's husband, (they had their business together, and, they are cousins.) Gary answered the phone and when I told him that I had breast cancer, he did not say anything. He knew when he felt the lump that it was not good. He asked me what we would do next. The question we all needed to know, and I was not waiting three days to find out. I told him we were on our way to find out.

I called my mom at work to give her the news. This was not the kind of information you want to tell your mother over the phone, but I had to. I told her I had breast cancer and Sandy and I were going to pick up the results. She said she wanted to come with us, so I told her we would pick her up at her house in one hour. When we picked my mom up, you could see she had been crying and I told her that it would be fine, she said, "It's not fine," you should not have to be going through this, you don't deserve it, and I told her "nobody deserves it."

When we arrived at the doctors office, (visibly shaken and upset) to get copies of my results, the nurse made a statement, about not jumping to any conclusions "It's just cancer she said." Sandy and I looked at each other and said, "JUST CANCER." We were horrified! You don't tell someone they have cancer and then say not to worry. I knew right then this was not going to be the doctor who was going to make decisions about my life. If the nurse was this shallow (then what does that say about the doctor?)

I called work and told my supervisor that I had breast cancer and I was not able to come back for the next couple of days. I needed to find out what to do next. She told me to take as much time as I needed, I was very pleased to hear that because she wasn't always the nicest person in the world. I asked her to please explain to the girls I worked with what was going on, because I left for lunch and never came back. I would call and update her as soon as I had more information. I knew it would be an emotional meeting since one of our other friends (Laura 43) was just diagnosed six months before me with breast cancer. She was out of work and undergoing chemotherapy and radiation treatments. There were five of us who became very close friends, (Christina, Donna, Laura, Katrina and Annie). We all were very upset when we were told about Laura's cancer and now they are being told about me. It was a bit frightening that two women in the same office developed breast cancer in a matter of six months. I was a little freaked out, was it something in the water, the air, the building. Something was not right about this office there had been several people diagnosed with different types of cancer all within a 2 year period.

I picked up the phone and called the one person I knew who could help; Dr. P., he was the one who order all of the initial testing. I prayed that he was working, when the receptionist told me he was, she put him on the phone, he had already read my results, he told me to come to his office immediately. He actually put his entire practice aside; he was so incredible, and cared about every one of his patients, he would have done that for anyone. I am so lucky to have a doctor as caring as him.

He sat with my mom, Sandy and I to explain what should be done next. We still had no idea how bad the cancer really was. He told me that he felt I would definitely have to have chemotherapy and radiation but I needed to see an oncologist. He recommended Dr. M., an oncologist out of town. Dr. P. explained that he was highly recommended and thought that I would receive the best care with him.

I remember sitting in the chair listening to what Dr. P., was saying but not absorbing it. My thoughts were all over the place. I was thinking about my son and husband. Sandy had a note pad with twenty questions written on it she was asking all the questions, and writing stuff down. I was crying and he asked me, "Why are you crying?" Is it because you are going to lose your hair? I said "yes." The fact that the chemo would make me sick was easier to accept then accepting the fact my hair was going to fall out.

The Pathology Report

Dr. P., then explained the type of cancer I had, it's called IDC-Invasive ductal carcinoma. Invasive means that it has "invaded" or spread to the surrounding tissues. It is "ductal" because the cancer began in the milk ducts-which are the "pipes" that bring milk from the lobules to the nipple. We all know what carcinoma is (cancer). Mine is "invasive" poorly differentiated duct carcinoma of unfavorable modified Bloom-Richardson grade 3. (9/9 Tubules= 3; Mitotic Activity =3; Nuclear Pleomorphism =3.)

Grade 3 cancer cells do not look like normal cells, they are fast growing. This is the worst grade of cancer anyone could have. The tumor was found in all four biopsy cores. Which meant that the cancer cells broke through the walls of the breast and could potentially spread into other parts of my body?

It is a very aggressive form of cancer for someone my age. ER-negative tumors are usually not affected by the levels of estrogen and progesterone in your body. The one time I wanted to hear the word "positive" may really mean something good, usually "positive" is bad. In my case I was "negative" not what the doctors wanted to see.{ My immunohistochemical (the scientific study of the way the immune system works in the body) studies demonstrated no nuclear staining for estrogen or progesterone receptor (ER negative, PR negative) my HER2/Neu was scored as 1+ and interpreted as negative.}

All of this medical terminology and I just want it explained in a way that I could understand. What does this all mean, will I live or die? What is my prognosis? That's what I really needed to hear, and of course no one can really answer those questions.

We still had to wait for some more of the biopsy results to come back and I needed to have the lump removed, before we would know the stage of my cancer.

I thanked Dr. P., for seeing us so fast and just taking the time out to care and place everyone else on hold to help me. Most doctors would have never done that.

Chapter Six

"Denial"

After a long exhausting day, we headed home to set up appointments. I needed an oncologist and a breast surgeon. Sandy helped by making all of the appointments from her cell phone. (I was in denial and went into the grocery store to get something to make for dinner) acting like it was just another day.

I now had to break the news to the rest of the family, but I wanted to wait until Gary came home from work, so I could explain to him first what was actually happening. When Gary came home I sat with him and showed him all of the results. I tired to explain to him in a way that he would understand. It all was a bit confusing.

I had Gary call his mom, who was watching Owen, and ask if she would bring Owen home for us. Then I called the rest of the family, so many people to call I was getting tired of talking about it. (My son was too young to understand what was happening which was a blessing.)

> "I have to say, I am very lucky to have such a loving husband, he is also suffering in his own way. He is an amazing, caring, generous, loving, man, I have been blessed to have him in my life. A lot of people forget about the spouse and child, when their loved one is stricken with this disease. I believe that they have been hit just as hard as I." They are suffering in there own way.

Feeling a bit confused, I think I was in denial about what was really happening. We dropped my mother off at her house and she was going to call my father at work he had no idea that my results came back positive. My mother, father, Dave and Sandy were coming to my house for dinner. We would sit and discuss my diagnosis. Then figure out a game plan.

I called my best friend Dawn who was working; when she answered the phone I explained to her that I had breast cancer. (We have been friends since junior high school.) It was very quiet on the other end, like everyone else was when I told them. Dawn asked me; "how could you be so calm?" I told her that I had to pull myself together for Gary and Owen. I cried all day and it was not the time to sit back and feel sorry for myself. I had breast cancer and there was nothing I could do to make it go away at this moment. I had to accept the fact I was sick and start to fight. I would not allow myself to break down in front of them. It was the last thing they needed to see. Dawn told me that she would stop by when she got home from work. Our friendship is very special, not only have we been best friends for over twenty years, we were pregnant together. Her daughter was born in August of 2000. My son was born in September 2000. We have a very special bond, which will last forever.

Sandy and I were able to get an appointment with a local oncologist the next day, May 22; their office was located in the lower Hudson valley.

We also made an appointment with Dr. M., the oncologist Dr. P., recommended. That appointment was set for May 26.

Chapter Seven

"Second Opinions Are Very Important."

When we went to see the local oncologist the doctors immediately wanted to put in a port a cath. Sandy and I looked at each other and said thanks but NO thanks. (I had NO clue what a port a cath even was, but I went with the flow, Sandy obviously new what it was. I trusted her to make that decision for me.) They also seemed to be very laid back and unconcerned. I wasn't feeling a connection. We definitely were not going to that oncologist. When we went to see Dr. M., we had to travel about fifty minutes south to get to his office, he is the doctor that Dr. P., recommended.

"Everything changed the day I met Dr. M."

At this point I was so tired, emotionally broken down, and overwhelmed, I couldn't even think straight. It still felt like a dream, I kept asking myself in my head *"why me" "why now,"* so many things were happening in my life and my families lives within the past two months, some where great and others were sad, how much more could go wrong in one family. It felt as if my whole world was crashing down right in front of me.

I felt so bad for my mom, she was devastated. I knew what was going through her mind, I was more afraid of her having a mental break down, then myself. I wished that she did not have to be going through this. I did not care about myself at the time, I worried about everyone else. Because if I die then my family will be left without me, they will be the ones suffering. "I just wanted to hold my son and my husband, and forget that this frightening nightmare has happened to us." I was hoping to go to sleep and wake up in the morning and it would all be a bad dream. When I woke up in the morning it wasn't just a bad dream, this was reality it was time to stand strong and fight.

I wasn't ready to die and leave my family and friends. My son, out of everyone, needed me the most.

Time Really Does Matter!

The breast surgeon I wanted to see was booked for six weeks; her office was located in Dutchess County. I couldn't wait a month, but I had no idea where to find a good breast surgeon. Sandy was making phone calls and appointments. Thankfully, she is very controlling when it comes to a crisis situation, and won't stop until she gets answers. I also needed to have a breast MRI, which we managed to get that done within the week at an Imaging center south from where I lived. We had to travel because, Dutchess county did not have a breast MRI machine as of yet.

At the Imaging center I met with the most remarkable radiologist. He and his staff were all very caring and understanding of my concerns. After the MRI he took us into his office and explained what he had seen on the films. He did see the tumor and informed us that the lymph nodes didn't look abnormal, but until they came out we would not know for sure. That was some positive news!

Chapter Eight

"Reality"

I finally met with Dr. M., the oncologist down the line and his nurse practitioner, Cindy. I remember Cindy came into the room first and looked at me, then walked back out of the room. A few seconds later she came back in and said "oh my God" I thought I was in the wrong room. This must be a mistake. When she sat down and looked over the films and biopsy results she turned to Sandy and me and said "Karen you know that you can die, right?" Talk about being blunt! I knew I was in the right place after meeting with her.

Dr. M. walked in the room with the biggest smile I have ever seen. He has a kind gentle soul he is like a big teddy bear, with a huge heart. I was so comfortable meeting the two of them I knew I would be safe in their care. These were the people who were going to safe my life.

Dr. M. gave me a treatment plan, which consisted of four rounds of Adriamycin and cytoxin and four rounds of Taxotere, then 33 sessions of radiation. Before I was able to start treatment the doctor needed to remove the tumor and make sure the cancer had not spread to my lymph nodes, find out the staging of my cancer, and make sure the cancer wasn't anywhere else in my body. This meant I had to have x-rays, a CAT scan, a bone scan, blood work, and a mug scan (which checked my heart to make sure it was strong enough for the Adriamycin.)

My first set of tests were done at the local hospital where Dr. M's office was located. He sent Sandy and me downstairs to the basement of this hospital where they did the CAT scan and x-rays. I felt like I was in the morgue, it was cold, gloomy and very unpleasant. We even had to sit in metal chairs, which were not at all comfortable. I felt bad for Sandy because she was pregnant, and she had to be uncomfortable, she never once complained. (We were down there for four hours.)

One of the nurses brought me out a white chalky looking drink, the doctors call it contrast. (Contrast lights up in your body if something is abnormal and not supposed to be there.) It did have some flavor but not much. I had to drink two liter size containers, it was horrible. I could barely get it down my throat. Sandy kept telling me to hold my nose, but that didn't work, I even tried to pour it into a small Dixie cup and drink it like a shot. Every time I took a sip I started to gag, my mouth was watering, my eyes were tearing, and I almost threw it all up. I knew I had to have these test to make sure the cancer wasn't anywhere else in my body. So I had no choice. I had to drink it and keep it down.

The Right Breast Surgeon

When I was finished downstairs, Dr. M., asked me to return to his office to finish our appointment, he asked if I had a breast surgeon yet and I told him that I needed to find one. The one that I was going to use was unable to see me for at least six weeks. (He couldn't believe that a surgeon would not see me for six weeks, with the type of results that I had, one more month without any type of treatment my cancer would have possibly spread, it was that aggressive.) He was so sweet and said "come with me, sweetie, I have the perfect person for you."

He walked Sandy and me through the halls of the hospital to one of the top breast surgeons in America.

I knew from the moment that I met him he would be the best surgeon for me.

He was very thorough with the breast exam. He asked me so many questions. One question he asked was if anyone in my immediate family had ever been diagnosed with breast cancer. I explained to him that my great grandmother was the only person that I knew who had breast cancer. He did not think that she was maternal to me because she was my mother's grandmother. With that being said he believed that all I needed to do was have a lumpectomy. Sandy and I asked about a partial mastectomy, he did not think that was necessary at this time.

When the breast surgeon suggested that I have a lumpectomy he also said he would be performing a sentinel node dissection, he wanted this done immediately.

He scheduled the surgery for May 30, 2003, a same day surgery. I was very pleased with how quickly Sandy and I managed to get all of this done, four weeks from finding the lump. "I just want this cancer to go away." I wanted it out of my body!

The girls that worked in his office were fantastic, very helpful, and caring. I was able to connect with the receptionist because she had told me that she had had breast cancer and had been cancer free for a few years. That was great to know that someone my age had beaten the disease. The other young woman took care of the insurance end of the paperwork and setting the appointments for surgery.

Chapter Nine

So Much Heartache
"May 29, 2003"

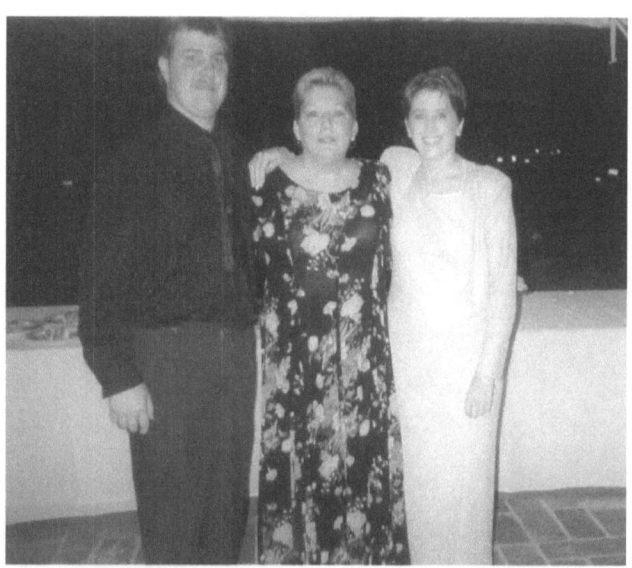

Aunt Kathy, David (my brother) and Karen

My family and I buried my aunt the day before my surgery. We had no time to mourn the death of her because I was diagnosed right in the middle of her illness. I was trying to help my cousins because they were only 18 and 21 when she died; they had been through so much heart ache with their mom over the years. This was the time that they both needed her the most. It was heart breaking to watch my cousins suffer so badly when she died. My mom and I had been suffering also, but we were distracted by my illness, we hadn't been able to mourn my aunt's death. I believe that God took her and not me because he has plans for me. It was not my time to go!

Lumpectomy Time

May 30th arrived and it was finally time to remove the cancerous tumor from my breast. I had been waiting patiently for the past four weeks. I just wanted this ugly, disgusting disease to leave my body. Sandy picked my mother and me up at my house and we set off to the hospital. We ended up getting there late because there had been an accident on RT-684, so we had to take a detour. We were not to sure how else to get to the hospital. We called a friend of Sandy's and she gave us directions from the Taconic, we actually crossed the same bridge two times. We were very confused, I think that the fact we all were so nervous about this surgery, none of us had our heads on straight.

We finally did arrive at the hospital only about forty five minutes late. The nurse told us that we were not the only ones running late, the doctor was too. Once I was signed in I was brought back to the pre op holding area. The nurse ran an IV line and started me on a saline drip she asked the typical questions they always asked. Once I was set and ready to go, my mom and Sandy came to sit with me. I was really scared about this surgery this was it this will tell all.

The doctor came over to see me before surgery. He wanted to go over everything that was going to happen in the operating room. He wanted to explain what he was going to do, then said, "Are you ready to roll?" I was so ready, I told him lets do this and get it done. I told my mom and Sandy see you soon they both hugged me and said good luck we love you. The surgeon told them he would take great care of me. The surgery will be about two hours.

Through the doors I went, it was very cold, and had this awful medicated smell, everything was white and silver. The nurse helped me onto the operating table, gave me a warm blanket, I was shaking it was so cold. The anesthesiologist injected me with something to relax me, the doctor said every thing would be just fine, he asked me about my son, he could see I was nervous, I told him my son wanted to be the next Tiger Woods, the next thing I remember I was asleep. I didn't even remember saying that.

During the surgery after removing the tumor the surgeon sent the sentinel node to pathology for a frozen section to see if the cancer spread to the lymph nodes. This way he would know if he had to remove any more nodes while I was still under anesthesia. The results came back negative, which meant the cancer had not spread to the lymph nodes. When I woke from surgery, my mom and Sandy were standing over me with big smiles on their faces and said "we finally received some good news, the frozen section was negative." Finally something good happened!

Everything from the start was such bad news that I was sure it was the end for me. I was so happy that none of my lymph nodes tested positive. Due to the size of the tumor this meant that my cancer was Stage 1. It was hard enough that my HER2/neu and ER, PR were all negative. I thought that would be good news, the doctors would have liked to see these results positive; I then would have been able to go on tamoxifen, a drug which inhibits the actions of estrogen

Once the final pathology report from my surgery came back and proved that the lymph nodes where clear, I started my treatment of chemo with Dr. M. The date was, June 10, 2003.

Chapter Ten

Chemotherapy Begins

The dreadful morning came for my first round of chemo I had to be there early. Gary had to be at work, so Sandy drove me and my mom to the hospital. The nurse called me back to have my bloods checked before I started treatment. This would be something that was done every time I came for a treatment. Once the doctor saw that all my blood work was in normal range, I was brought into the treatment room. This room was filled with reclining chairs and nurses taking care of other patients having their chemo.

Cindy, (the doctors nurse practitioner) would be the one giving me my very first treatment. She sat down next to me and we started talking, she had no idea that Sandy was pregnant, but during conversation with her it came up and Cindy kicked her out of the treatment room (in a very nice way). The toxic fumes would not be good for her since she was in her first trimester, but my mom was allowed to be with me, Thank God, because I was scared to death. I tried to tell Sandy to stay home but she wasn't having it. She had to be there. I wanted her to take care of herself because she was about two months pregnant. It wasn't just about her anymore; she had a baby growing inside of her who needed her to be healthy.

I remember sitting in a chair with a blanket in the cold treatment room, why are the rooms always cold? It must be because of germs.

It was quiet and everyone looked so sick, all I could hear were beeping noises from the IV machines. No one was really talking, just the nurses. I was looking at all the other people, not just women but men too, being hooked up to their IV machines, receiving chemotherapy in all different forms. I was the youngest person in the room, I was so scared, I had NO idea what to expect. I remember thinking to myself, how many of these people are going to survive. I just started to cry, "This shouldn't be happening." So many things go through your mind when you are faced with death. Trying to stay positive and focused is very hard.

Cindy started my IV, gave me something to calm my nerves, and started a saline drip. She explained what some of the side effects were going to be. It was so much to comprehend; I had to have steroids, nausea medicine, anxiety meds, shots etc. With so much to remember, my mom had to write things down for me because I couldn't even focus.

It's very important to have someone with you at all appointments to help you understand what is being said, there was always something else I had to remember. Every time I had to have treatments the nurses had to place an IV in my left hand, because I didn't have a port. My veins were not the greatest veins in the world; the nurses had trouble every time. When they stick that long needle into the top of your hand it feels like it is hitting the bone. It hurts so badly.

I had to learn how to give myself a needle for the day after chemo, this way I wouldn't have to drive all the way there for just a five minute visit. This was an injection called Neulasta; it helps level out the white cells, it reduces risk of fever and low white blood cell count.

About half an hour after the saline drip, Cindy started the steroids and Cytoxan; this would drip very slowly to make sure I wouldn't have an allergic reaction. (Plus this was my very first treatment.) Once that was half way through Cindy sat next to me and started to explain the AC;

Adriamycin-Doxorubicin, "anthracycline-antibiotic" actually looked like red fruit punch but thicker. This was in a big round tube, (there were two of them,) Cindy said she was going to start to push the liquid through my IV into my veins very slowly. This was so toxic that it would cause tissue damage and blistering if it escapes from the vein. These side effects of the Adriamycin include nausea, vomiting, fatigue, hair loss, heart problems, bladder problems, sores in the mouth and your urine turns red, often mistaken for blood.

Cyclophosphamide-Cytoxan was the poison that would eventually make my hair, eyebrows, and eyelashes fall out, take away my appetite, make me fatigued, and stop my menstrual cycle.

What this does is kill all the cells in your body since the chemotherapy doesn't know the difference between "normal" and "cancerous." The normal cells will grow back. It takes months for a cell count to become normal again after having this type of chemotherapy treatment.

The doctor said my hair would fall out about seventeen days after the first treatment.

About six hours later I was finally done with my first round of chemotherapy I had only seven more to go. I was mentally drained and anxious, waiting for something to happen. I heard the stories and saw the movies of people who get sick after chemo so this is kind of what I was expecting. I took my nausea meds every day and my steroids the day before treatment, during treatment, and the day after treatment. Because my cancer was so aggressive, my treatments were scheduled for every two weeks instead of every three.

By the third day after my first treatment, I started to feel some of the side effects: a little nausea, and a lot of irritability, I could not sit still or lie down for long because I felt like I had things crawling on me. I hated this feeling but I thought if this is all then I can handle it.

As the week passed I started to feel okay, not great, but able to go about my normal routine, which includes taking care of my son, husband, and the household chores. I knew that things would only start to get worse so I had to get as many things done around the house and with Owen before it was too late. I took family medical leave from work, because I was too sick to do the kind of work they needed me to do. It was summer time I wanted to take Owen outside to play, but being in the sun made me feel very sick to my stomach. Gary works outside for a living so when he got home from work the last place he would want to be is outside in the heat. Gary and Owen would play with his hot wheel cars, and Owen and I would color a lot.

I went for treatments every other Tuesday at 9:00am. Owen would stay with a family member every time I went for chemo. My treatments were always about five to six hour days. I would always get a turkey sandwich on white bread and a big bottle of water to bring with me to eat during my treatment, and then I would drop Owen off to who ever had been watching him that day. It was so hard leaving him in the morning knowing that he may not have a lot of time left with me. What if something happens to me during my treatment? This made me so angry, why me, he is so young and he just doesn't understand why his mommy is so sick. I felt guilty that he would be missing so much time with me, I wouldn't be able to do the things that moms do with their kids. I wasn't able to have him around other children because I couldn't risk getting sick with an infection. I couldn't run around outside with him because it was to hot and I was unable to be in the direct sun light. These are all things little kids are supposed to be able to do with their moms. I felt horrible and guilty for being so sick. We had to pretty much stay secluded in the house.

During my second treatment I wasn't as anxious because I knew what to expect. It was very hard to sit in the treatment room with all of the other people who were sick (wondering what was wrong with them) or (how long they had to live.) They all weren't there for the same type of cancer, some had breast cancer, lung cancer, bone cancer, skin cancer, and one woman even had brain cancer. It was so depressing. I almost felt guilty for only having stage 1T cancer, I had a very good survival rate. (Everyone would tell me not to, worry it's only stage 1, well, let me tell you something, it's still cancer and cancer kills.)

Chapter Eleven

"Hair" It Goes!

Dr. M. would check my white cells every time I went in for treatment to make sure that they were in a normal range so I would be able to receive treatment that day. He came into the treatment room to check on me and say hello, he tugged on my hair, looked at me and asked me "did any fall out yet?"

I said "nope not yet," hoping maybe he would be wrong and it would not fall out.

Tuesday night after I got home from chemotherapy I sat with my son and started to explain that mommy was sick and would have to have special medicine to help make me feel better. Since he was only two and a half, he had no clue about what really was going on. I told him that in a few days mommy's hair would fall out and I would look like daddy. Owen said in his sweet little innocent voice, "Daddy no hair, Mommy hair." I asked him if he wanted to play a game and see who could pull out the most. I was trying to make a game of it so he would not be afraid. He immediately started pulling on my hair.

The next morning I woke up and noticed a little hair on my pillow: I knew it was time, boy was the doctor right! It was seventeen days to be exact, when my hair started falling out. It would come out in clumps, especially in the shower. That first day was the hardest, running my hands through my head and it falling out in hands full, I have never cried so hard in my life. I locked myself in the bathroom because I didn't want anyone to hear or see me cry. It was hard enough for Gary and Owen to see me look like this, I wanted everyone else to think I was okay; I didn't want them to worry about me all the time. Looking in the mirror and I don't even recognize myself anymore, is this what someone with cancer looks like? This can not be me, I felt like a stranger in my own house. This is where it all began, who am I?

Once my hair started to fall out it did not stop. I had a hard time with shaving it because I did not want to be bald, but my husband said he rather see me bald then with strands of hair missing, because that made me look worse. So I called Sandy she and her husband came over. I asked Gary if he wanted to shave the rest of my hair off, but he wanted no part of that. So, Sandy took Gary's shaver and we sat on the back deck and she shaved the rest of my hair off. I was devastated; I could not believe my hair was gone. It definitely put everything into prespective about this horrifying disease. Owen thought it was cool that both his parents were now bald. We tried to convince him to shave his head but he did not want to look like us. I couldn't blame him.

It felt so weird to be bald, but thank God it was summer because it was a lot cooler being bald then having hair. Now I had to go out and buy some bandanas, I wasn't crazy about wearing a wig. I didn't mind wearing baseball caps.

The next day I went to one of my hair dressers, and asked him if he could clean up my bald head. He was shocked when I walked in with no hair, since two months before he was styling it for Sandy's wedding. "What happened?" Did you have a bad hair day? We laughed!

I said, "No I have breast cancer".

He looked at me and said, "Oh my God, I'm so sorry to hear that."

I told him not to be sorry, it is what it is, but can you please clean up my bald head. I had dark patches all over we hadn't used a professional shaver so it didn't give me a clean shave. He started to laugh and said "come with me." I know he wanted to cry, it was written all over his face. He was so nervous, I don't think he ever had a client walk into the salon with no hair and tell him they had cancer, and needed help. The day I went into the salon, it was a weekend and it was full of people. Every one was looking at me when I took off my baseball cap. My hair dresser asked me if I wanted to go somewhere else more private. I told him no, I have to get used to people looking at me and wondering what's wrong, I wasn't embarrassed!

Although everyone said how beautiful I looked bald, I knew they were all just trying to make me feel better. Come on now, women should have hair.

That evening, after the hair salon episode, I called my regular hair dresser, Jennifer. Although we had been friends for thirteen years, I hadn't seen her in a while because she had been out of work for a while. She was actually back to work when I called. When she picked up the phone I said to her, "Jennifer don't be mad at me I haven't been coming in because I have been going to Antonino; he did my hair for my friends wedding. Plus, I was trying to let it grow."

She said; "Karen you know me better then that, as long as he is doing a good job."

I said; "oh by the way, I have breast cancer and I am bald anyway!" When I didn't hear anything on the other end, I said "Jennifer, are you there?" she sounded like she was going to cry, I said I will beat this, but I have along road a head of me. She told me that she would take me for a wig when I was ready. I told her I already tried one and I didn't like the way it looked or felt. I just felt like everyone knew I was wearing one. I wasn't hiding the fact I had cancer so why should I bother being uncomfortable.

Chapter Twelve

Hope, Fight, and Courage

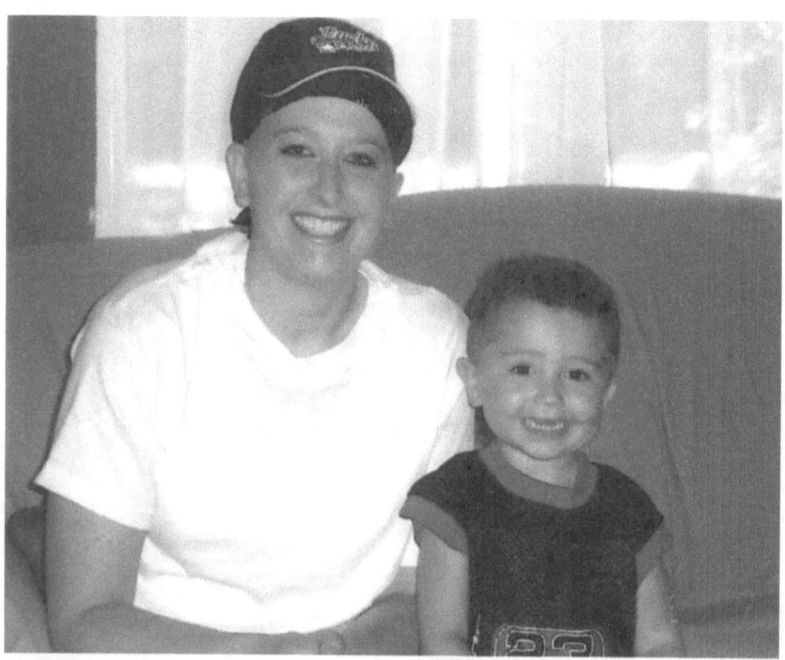

Karen and Owen

It was a Sunday evening I woke up in the middle of the night not feeling well. I was throwing up and when I looked in the bathroom mirror I saw for the first time, a sick person. I looked as if I was going to die. I was bald, pale, and had bags under my eyes and my face looked fat and round from all the steroids I had to take. I started to cry and could not believe this was really happening to me. The hardest part about being diagnosed with cancer is accepting the fact that you are sick. What did I do to deserve this? Why did I get cancer? As the weeks went by, the sicker I became. There were days I could not even get out of bed, but I had too, I have a young son who needed his mother. That is what I said to myself everyday, I never worried about me I was always worrying about everyone else around me. How is my husband dealing with this? What are my parents thinking? My own brother was so upset he could not even come to see me. This hurt me a lot, but I could understand. (I couldn't image how he and the rest of my family were feeling. They had to see me suffering.) What happens if I die? I started thinking where I wanted to be buried, what I wanted to wear in my casket, I didn't even have a "Will", "I better get one done," "what happens to Owen if something happens to Gary"? I was starting to plan my funeral, that way Gary wouldn't have to worry about anything. It would have been all taken care of. How will Owen and Gary survive without me? This just broke my heart every time I looked at the both of them.

I would go to bed every night and pray to God that I would wake up in the morning.

I knew that I had to beat this terrible disease, I needed to be strong and positive, and hope and fight with everything I had. I was not going to leave my family and friends and let this disease get me.

For God sakes, my father just buried his mother, my mother just buried her sister and their precious daughter could be dying from cancer-I was not going to be next.

"This all happened in 2 months!!!"

Every morning I made myself get up, and eat, and take care of Owen, it was so hard especially when I felt as if I had been struck with the flu, but ten times worse. Some days I was so weak that I could barely even walk, it was hard taking care of a small child and my self but I was too stubborn to ask for help. I felt as if I were already bothering too many people. My friend Dawn would bring over coolatas from Dunkin Donuts. I was so sick to my stomach that it was hard to keep anything down. I needed to stay hydrated, plus she knew how much I loved them.

"Sandy was pregnant and needed to take care of her, I felt like I took the joy out of what should have been the most exciting time of her life. She couldn't even enjoy being pregnant. I think there were times when she forgot she was even pregnant."

My husband was working so hard, he is self-employed so if he does not work then there is no money. Since I was on disability through work, I had to pay for my health insurance. What a joke that was! We counted on Gary's money to pay the bills, and we now didn't just have household bills, but also medical bills too.

Most of my family and friends were very helpful, Thank God; because by my fourth treatment I was so sick I just wanted to die. Four rounds were done with four more to go. I would actually start to feel sick right before I had to leave for treatment. The anticipation of having someone pump poison through my body just disgusted me.

Every week that I didn't have chemo I had to have blood work. My mother would take me to the laboratory, which was about five minutes away from where I lived. I was constipated from the treatments and so sick to my stomach. I walked in the door to have my blood drawn and there were so many people sitting there waiting. "I could not sit there and wait with all those people." I couldn't afford to get sick. Not feeling so good that day, I looked at my mother and said, "I can't do this right now," as I ran out of the building, my mother grabbed Owen's hand and followed me. I started throwing up all over the parking lot, people were coming in and out of the building, and I was so embarrassed. Owen asked my mother, "Why is mommy throwing up?"

"Is she okay?"

I heard my mother say to him, she will be fine honey; mommy just has a little tummy ache.

Summer Heat

It was now August, the hottest time of the year. I was preparing to start the next part of my chemotherapy, Docetaxel—[brand name: Taxotere] I had to have four cycles of this poison.

"This drug would be the hardest on my body." The doctors had to prepare me for the painful side effects that I was about to experience.

Taxotere kills cancer cells by stopping their growth. It can also make it hard for cancer cells to repair themselves. It stops the cancer cells from separating into two new cells. This was administered through my IV. It's a liquid form and drips (infusion) into the vein. The side effects are fatigue, nausea, some hair loss, headaches, aching muscles, and cough, abdominal cramps, nerve damage, problems with hands and feet. Your bones hurt as your bone marrow makes blood cells.

It was true-this chemo did all of the above; It made every bone in my body hurt from head to toe. It hurt so badly that I could not even move my head, forget about touching my skin. I just wanted all of this to be over. Night time was the hardest; I had trouble sleeping because of the pain. I never wanted to wake Gary because I felt bad bothering him since he had to get up to go to work. I would go down stairs and sit in the living room and just cry. I never wanted him to see me in pain. I would sit in the chair and try not to move. I would think to myself a lot and ask God to please just take me because I could not take it anymore. One night about 3:00am in the morning I was in so much pain I called my mom and my best friend Dawn to come over and sit with me. Dawn was another one of my friends who was always there for me. She would come over and just sit with me, take Owen to the play ground with her daughter. She even drove me to one of my chemo appointments.

Another night I called Sandy and asked her to come over because I had such bad chest pains, I thought I was having a heart attack. This was from the Taxotere. I was so scared I wanted her to take me to the hospital. I knew if I went to the hospital then I would have been admitted and I couldn't put that burden on anyone. Our lives had been torn upside down and I couldn't expect everyone to stop what they were doing to take care of me.

"I am so glad God did not listen to me."

I started to develop neuropathy in my hands and feet, and to this day I still have it, almost five years later. The doctor tells me that I'm that rare case who will have neuropathy for the rest of my life.

Chapter Thirteen

Owen Turns Three
"Happy Birthday"

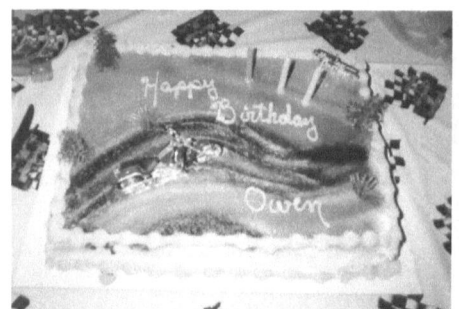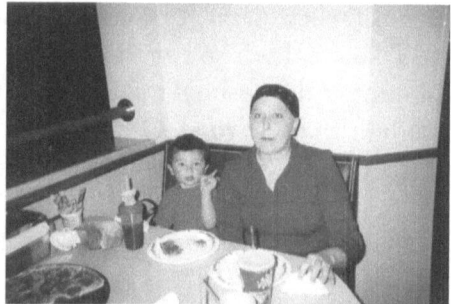

Owen Maneri and Mommy; Owen's Birthday Cake

September 10, 2003, Owen turned three today. Gary and I were planning a family party at our house, with our family and friends. I wanted to do something special for Owen because with everything that was going on in our lives, I felt like he was pushed aside. I was feeling sicker the further into my treatments. Since his party was not going to be until the weekend, I decided to take Owen to Chucky Cheeses. He wanted to go so bad. He always asked if we could go there. I always made excuses why we couldn't go, all the kids running around screaming and crying wasn't my cup of tea. This time I made an exception I packed a bag, with my medicine and water and off we went to Chucky Cheese. He was so excited. We arrived when they first opened, that way there would not be too many people. I asked my mother-in-law if she wanted to come with us. I didn't feel comfortable being by myself and since Gary was working he was unable to go. We sat down and ordered a pizza and something to drink. I took Owen around to play all the games. It was so nice to see him having fun. "I was having horrible hot flashes, and started to feel sick." After about two hours we handed in his tickets and he picked out his prizes. By the time we arrived home both Owen and I we're exhausted. So we took a nap until Gary came home from work.

It was the end of September. I finally finished the last round of chemotherapy and I was thrilled, but scared. It may sound silly but when you are having chemo, you feel safe because you know that the drug is killing off all the cells, but when you are finished, you get an overwhelming feeling wondering, "what if it comes back"!

I made baskets filled with herbal teas, willow tree angels, tea cups, candy, and cookies. I brought the baskets with me to my last round of chemo and handed them to all four of the nurses that treated me during chemo. "They truly were my guardian angels." I wanted them to feel appreciated.

Radiation Begins

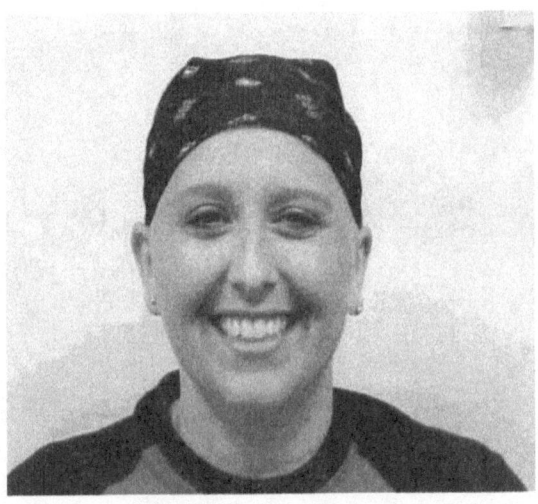

Me at first radiation

October finally arrived and the next part of my treatment started, radiation, again it was time to meet another set of doctors, with another set of opinions. I needed to have thirty three doses of radiation-every day except for Saturday and Sunday. Before you can start you have to be marked with small tattoos in the diseased area, (it does not really hurt you cannot even see the marks.) Once the radiation starts, it takes about one hour to finish. You have to wear a cotton hospital gown and you lie on a table, while the doctors aim this huge machine at the affected area. This machine marks the area with a red beam of light you do not even feel anything. The side effects start about one week after the first dose, you start to feel tired and you develop sunburn in the area of radiation, for which the doctor gives you a medicated cream to help heal the area.

At this point, I felt better because my hair had started to come in. My head looked like a big fat peach, it felt like one too! I was able to drive myself to my appointments which made me feel better. I didn't have to depend on anyone. I still had to find someone to sit with Owen when I went because he was unable to be there with me. Again, I had to drop him off to my mother-in-law and of course he cried every time. "When he cried I cried," I hated this feeling. Every day my anxiety got worse, I was tired of upsetting my family.

Happy Halloween
"Trick or Treat"

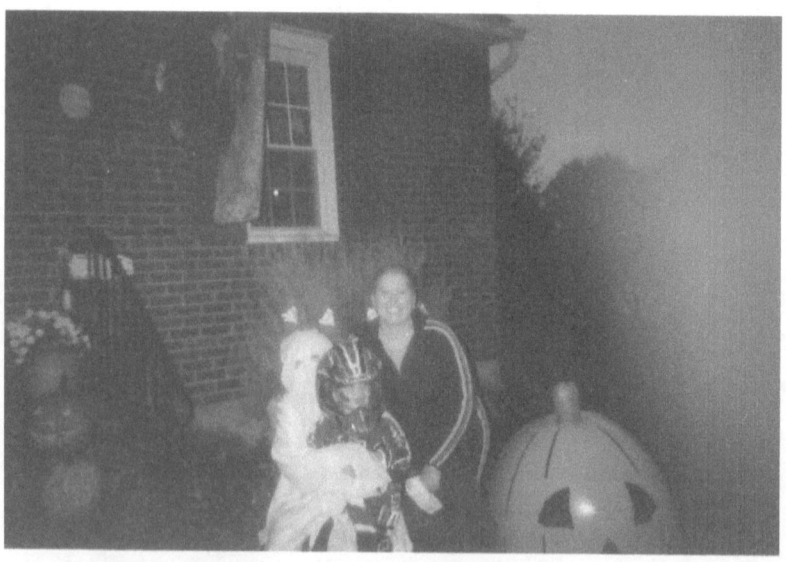

Owen and Mommy

It was a very exhausting month and a half, every day the same routine. I was still unable to go into public places due to risk of infection. My immune system still wasn't strong enough to handle an infection, It was definitely flu season and every one I knew was sick.

Halloween was coming up and Owen was three years old and was very excited to go out trick or treating. Every other year he had no interest in Halloween at all. He did not even want to give candy out. This year he wanted to dress up as a dirt bike rider. I was hoping he would want to stay home and hand out candy, "but he didn't!" It was one of the different fazes he was in. When the day came Gary and I took him out for a while and it was so nice to see him smiling and having so much fun.

"I just wanted to go home, I was tired and my feet were swollen."

I needed to see this and enjoy him as much as possible because I never knew when and if this disease would take me from him.

The Baby Shower

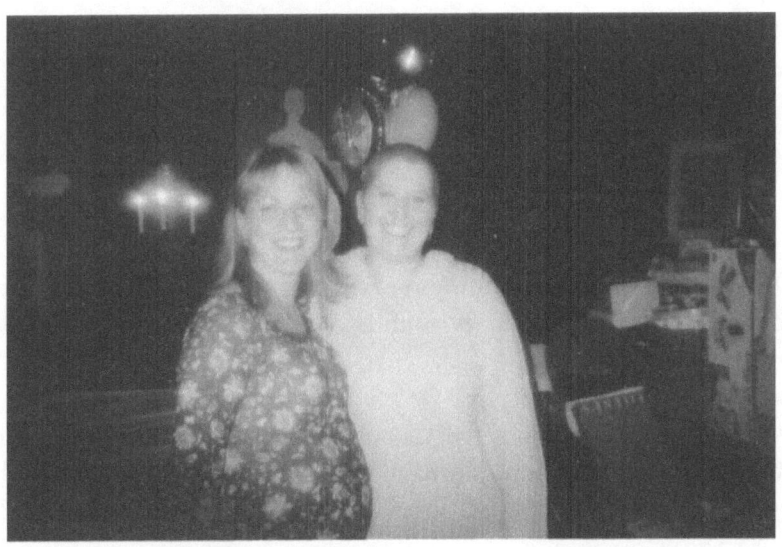

Sandy and Karen at the Baby Shower

Sandy's due date in January was getting closer. I didn't think she was going to make it to her due date. She was huge, for someone so small, I couldn't believe how big she was, if you were to tap her on the back she would have probably tipped over, she was so off balance.

Her sister in laws and I decided to give her a baby shower, I was extremely tired from all of the radiation, so I couldn't really help out too much. I did however write out all of the invitations and then mail them out. We planned it for November 9th at a local restaurant, always so much easier, no clean up on our end.

It was a beautiful day but a little cold; "it was November," my hair started coming in very slowly, it was fuzzy and dark; I was still uncertain about having hardly any hair and being around so many people, but everyone made be feel really comfortable. Sandy had invited about sixty people, she knew about the shower because it was much easier with everything that was going on in our lives at the time.

At the shower Sandy received a ton of gifts, (earlier she found out she was having a boy!!!) The shower was beautiful; the food was fantastic, (even though I had no taste buds) another side effect of chemotherapy. Her friends and family were all there. It was nice to have something fun to look forward too. By the end of the day I was wiped out, I was still having radiation and it just exhausted me.

I believe that her baby was one big reason why I made it though one of the toughest times of my life.

"Everything was so black for me with my diagnosis there
was a bright ray of hope in her pregnancy."

We would soon be welcoming a new little one to the family, I felt like this baby was part mine, it may sound crazy but he was with us through everything, from day one.

Sandy and I talked everyday, we spent almost everyday together except when she worked. We had a special bond, one that could not be broken. Because her husband and my husband are first cousins, our boys would be second cousins. I was excited because Owen is an only child he needs young cousins to grow up with.

"Owen does have other cousins, D.J. (David) is thirteen, Miranda is ten, Angelena is Three, Michael is two, and Jenna Marie is one years old. (Daniel would be closest in age.)"

When the last session of radiation came I felt a BIG sigh of relief. It was December, and it was cold. I still didn't have a lot of hair. I couldn't wait to put all of this behind me and try to get back into some kind of normal routine and to eventually get back to work. I lost seven months of my life with my son and husband it makes me so angry that I had to lose any time with the both of them. I felt like I was missing out on so many things with my family, while trying to battle this deadly disease.

Chapter Fourteen

Christmas Eve
"Merry Christmas"

December 24, 2003, rolled around. What a long seven months it had been. The mail carrier knocked on the door; she had something for me to sign. (She was always so nice to me and my family, every day she would ask how I was feeling.) When I opened the envelop, I saw a letter from my employer, I had been out on disability for the past six months when I read the letter it was telling me that I was "FIRED." I could not believe what I was reading; they fired me because I was sick and could not come to work. Wasn't there a law for that?

My boss said when I was able to come back to work I would be able to re apply for my position. I could not believe this was happening on Christmas Eve, no less, Happy New Year I said to myself. If getting cancer and being bald were not bad enough, I now lost my job. How in the world was I supposed to get another job when I had no hair, eyebrows, or eyelashes? I looked like an alien from another planet and to top it off I was thirty pounds over weight. Would anyone hire me? I didn't even look like a woman I thought to myself. I am a cancer patient!

I now became more depressed. I secluded myself in my house: I didn't want to talk to anyone. I started to feel sorry for myself, which was something that I didn't want to happen.

"It finally occurred to me that if I didn't get some help things would only get worse. I knew now it was time to see a therapist. Everyone one else in my life had to be tired of listening to me complain about how crappy I felt and why my bones hurt, something always hurt. I felt like a hypochondriac, I guess I had every right to feel that way, but I didn't want it to consume my life. Don't get me wrong I was thankful that the cancer was gone but I hated the fact that I was 34 years old and was limited as to what I could do and how I felt. The doctors explained how I would feel when I was going through treatment, but no one prepared me for what I would feel like after the treatments stopped."

Christmas Day

"2003"

It was early Christmas morning and Owen woke Gary and me up at about 6:00am. He was so excited about seeing all the presents that Santa Clause brought him. He was afraid to go downstairs by himself. I rolled out of bed and we headed downstairs. "His face lit up like a Christmas tree." The presents were every where. This was the first Christmas that he actually could understand the concept of Santa Clause. "Gary and I wanted to make it a very special year." Owen had seen a lot of sadness in our home over the past seven months and we needed to make it joyful for him. My whole family was coming over this year to celebrate. My mom and I were cooking at my house; I didn't want to run around to everyone else like we usually did. I wanted to be comfortable in my own home. We had a house full of friends and family we loved. My cousins came over, this would be their first Christmas without their Mother. Sandy and Dave, and Sandy's parents were over too. It was a very joyful day.

"Now this is what Christmas is all about." "Peace Love and Happiness."

Happy New Year 2004!
"It's a Boy!"

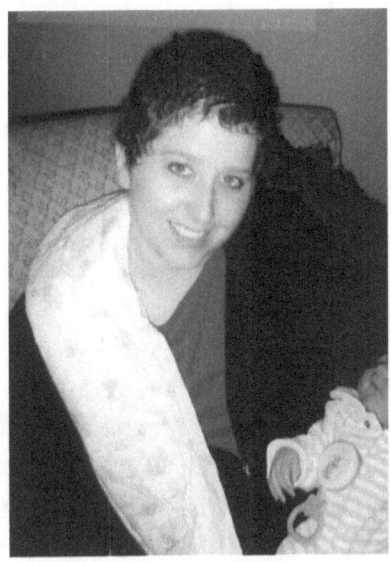

Karen and Daniel

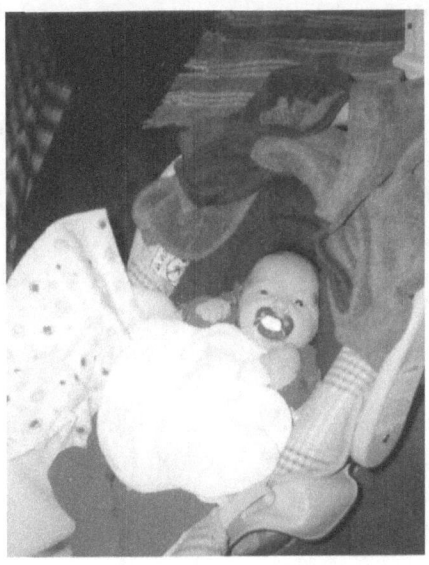

Daniel

It was now 2004; I was hoping to start the New Year off in better spirits. I knew this meant I had to try to overcome what had happened to my family and me throughout the past year.

Soon there would be a brand new baby. Sandy asked me if I would be in the delivery room with her, and of course I said yes, what a wonderful gift that was. The time came—it was January 10th and I received the call from her about 10:00pm she said "Karen I think my water broke, I can't even get off the toilet."

I told her I would be right there. Her mom met me at Sandy's house, Dave was getting ready and I helped Sandy put something more comfortable on. Her contractions were only three minutes apart. I thought for sure we would not make it to the hospital in time. It seemed like forever to get there. I rode with Patty, Sandy's mom, and when we arrived at the hospital the nurse brought us into her room. She told us she was only two centimeters dilated. We all were shocked; we knew it was going be a long night.

This day seemed like forever from when she first found out she was pregnant. We had so many distractions with my illness that before we knew it the baby was on its way. It was a long night and Sandy had a very hard delivery, seventeen hours of hard labor, and no sleep. I couldn't believe that I was experiencing this beautiful moment. I have never seen someone give birth before. "It is so different when you are the one pushing the baby out."

Finally after about two hours of pushing, out came Daniel, weighing in at 8lbs 12oz, it was no wonder she had so much trouble pushing him out. A beautiful healthy baby boy, he was huge and beautiful. I cried so hard I couldn't believe this little angel baby was finally here. He shared so many conversations, and tears with us along the way. It was about time that something so special and beautiful came into the world and I was still around to see it. I couldn't wait to hold him and just love him like he was my own. Sandy and Dave asked Gary and I to be Daniels Godparents we accepted with open arms.

Scan Time

Now that my treatments were finished I had to have another round of CAT scans, bone scans, and a mug scan for my heart because of the AC (chemo) treatment.

"This is the hard part, not knowing what they may find".

I didn't realize how many appointments that I had gone to, until I was finished. There is always a follow up appointment, weekly blood tests, monthly doctor appointments, and not just with one doctor.

"I went to over 200 doctor appointments in one year."

Sandy drove me to my appointment. It was time for my first CAT scan and bone scan since my diagnosis. I had to drink that disgusting contrast; I could barely get it down again. I started to feel sick to my stomach. When it was time for the CAT scan I was injected with another form of contrast. This, when injected makes your whole body feel warm, like you may pee yourself and you get a metal taste in your mouth.

I had had enough by this time, between all the chemo and radiation; I was tired of going for tests and scans. I knew it had to be done so I had to just accept it.

After the CAT scan I had a bone scan scheduled at the hospital around the corner, both tests in the same day. When I arrived at the hospital I went upstairs to nuclear testing and was injected with another type of contrast that was used for the bone scan. By this time I started to have diarrhea it was horrible. I was sick to my stomach; I could not even eat anything. I was miserable! I still had to lye on the table for forty minutes and have that scan done. I prayed that I wouldn't throw up all over the place.

On our way home I started to feel really sick, I remember Sandy who never drives over the speed limit driving so fast to get me home. Daniel was only a few weeks old and fast asleep in his car seat. I got really quiet and all of a sudden I said; "I think I'm going to be sick," she, being a nurse, grabbed a basin bucket (this is what they give to throw up in at the hospital), out from under her car seat and handed it to me. She was trying to pull off the road and suddenly I started vomiting in this little basin bucket, trying not to get all over the car. She pulled off the side of the highway; I jumped out and vomited all over the ground. After about ten minutes I felt a little better, we both started to laugh. (I couldn't believe she had that basin in her car, leave it to Sandy).

I will never forget that day; it was at exit 18 on Route 84. Now every time I pass that exit I just laugh to myself.

Chapter Fifteen

Who am I?

Before breast cancer, I was very out going, social, and self assured, after breast cancer that all changed. I had nothing left inside of me to give; it took my mind and spirit. I became a very angry person inside. I was now on a mission to find out why this had happened to me. I never had a mean bone in my body and I hated that I felt angry all the time. I had no known family history of breast cancer except for my great grandmother on my mother's side. She had breast cancer in the late sixties. Although she never had chemotherapy she had a bilateral mastectomy and she survived 20 more years. When she did pass on it wasn't from cancer but from old age. This was not considered family history to me because she was not maternal to me; she was my mother's grandmother. "I never could quite figure that out." A friend of mine mentioned genetic testing, and suggested that I be tested to make sure it wasn't hereditary. I spoke to Gary and asked him if he thought that genetic testing would be beneficial to me. "He agreed that I should look into it". I started to do my own research on the computer, and after extensive research I knew the only way to find out where this horrible disease came from was if I was tested.

Genetic Testing
"I need to know"

At my next visit with Dr. M, I decided to ask him if he could run some blood work to see if I had this gene. I explained that I had done some research on genetic testing and I thought that I would definitely benefit by having this blood test. He didn't think it would come back positive, and he pretty much said to me he was sure it would be negative. He decided to run the test anyway if that's what would make me feel better. He knew how obsessive I was when it came to my health, so he wasn't going to deny me this opportunity to find out. He told me that these results must stay confidential and I should not tell anyone. This meant all my doctors; none of them were able to know the results. (If my insurance company were to find out then they could discriminate and possibly drop me from my insurance.)

The blood test was called Brca Analysis 1 and 2; the results would take about four to six weeks to come back, so Doctor M. wanted me to make my next appointment in a month. I was on a very short leash with all my doctors because of the aggressiveness of the cancer I had, and my age.

I made my appointment for the beginning of April 2004, my mom decided to come along with me so I was not by myself. Moms are always there when you need them and it's nice to have someone else with you so you don't feel so alone. Every time I went to an appointment by myself I received bad news. When Dr. M., came into the room he gave me a big hug, as he always did, and pinched my cheeks. He told me how beautiful I was. I just rolled my eyes and said;

"Beautiful? How anyone can look beautiful looking like this? I look horrible but thanks anyway." He sat there with me and my mom and said; "I have your results and I must say I was very surprised." I looked at my mom and we knew right then I was getting some more bad news. "Your blood work came back positive for Brca Analysis 1, and Brca Analysis 2 was inconclusive".

No one said a word; I could hear my mom start to cry. She tried so hard to hide it; we could not believe this was happening.

Now, this did not mean that the cancer was back it just meant that I had a mutation and cancer could strike me at anytime. Not everyone has this gene. It is hereditary, and my risk factor was an 87% chance of reoccurrence in the next five years in my breasts, ovaries, colon or prostate, (Thank God I don't have a prostate.) The good news was I had options that meant I could have a hysterectomy to avoid ovarian cancer, and a bilateral mastectomy to avoid breast cancer again. I knew if I did not do something that I would one day be sitting right back in that treatment room with cancer and no hair. That was not an option to me.

I went home and sat down with Gary so we could talk about what we wanted to do next. (I knew what I wanted, but I needed to hear from him what he was feeling.) There were a lot of pros and cons involved in these types of surgery. I felt this was not just my decision, I wanted his input, (we were a team), I was sure he would have concerns. He said what ever I chose he would support me 100%. So I chose the only option that seemed right for me and my family. I opted for the full hysterectomy and bilateral mastectomy with immediate reconstruction. The only concern my husband had was that I not wake up without breasts, he was not sure I could handle looking at myself like that, nor could he. I was already depressed enough that I had lost my hair and self-image, now I was going to have no breasts, (not real ones) and no female organs. My next question was how I explain this to my doctors, since Dr, M., suggested that I not tell any one in the health care field that I had this test done, because if it is in my medical files and the insurance company finds out they could drop me. This really made no sense to me because the insurance company offered to pay for the test. I scheduled an appointment to see Dr. P., my gynecologist he was the first one I wanted to see, I knew I could talk to him like a friend and not a patient and he would understand and do whatever it took to help me. I told him that I was more afraid of getting ovarian cancer then breast cancer. I actually was afraid that I may already have ovarian cancer, research showed that many women who had been diagnosed with breast cancer and tested positive with the brca gene had already had early stage ovarian cancer by the time they had a hysterectomy. He sent in something to my insurance company for authorization for a super cervical hysterectomy, everything would come out except for my cervix. This was for sexual reasons, "I am only 34" I still have sexual needs.

Once we had the insurance approval, surgery was scheduled for May 7, 2004. This is a major surgery which requires a few nights stay at the hospital. Now that this date was scheduled, it was time to see the breast surgeon. I made an appointment with Dr. C., to have a consult about a mastectomy. I went in with Sandy and we spoke to the doctor about a bilateral mastectomy with immediate reconstruction. He asked me "why would you want to have such an invasive surgery, especially when your cancer was early stage and no lymph nodes were affected?" My response to Dr. C., was, "if I could talk to you off the record then I will be able to tell you. If not, then I will have to lie." He said of course you can talk to me. "I said" Well, I tested positive for Brca 1'. He replied well that explains everything. 'We will get you scheduled as soon as possible.' He then asked if I had a plastic surgeon, I said I did not, so he referred me to doctor at a local hospital. When I told him that I was having a hysterectomy on May 7, he suggested that we wait at least eight weeks after that surgery before we start the other. They both are very invasive and each had long recovery periods plus the hysterectomy would put me in complete menopause, which I was not looking forward to, but after what I had just been through I figured it would be a piece of cake. Dr. C. scheduled my surgery for July 12, 2004. Now I had to see the plastic surgeon and figure out what type of reconstruction would be best for me.

Decisions, Decisions, Decisions!

I originally wanted to have skin sparing reconstruction with implants because it wasn't so invasive. Cindy, Dr. M.'s NPA told me not to let the doctors talk me into having a tram flap; (I didn't even know what a tram flap was.) **Tram** stands for (transverse rectus abdominis myocutaneous flap) a muscle located in the lower abdomen. They take your skin, fat and muscles and reconstructed new breasts, it sounded so painful. The tissue is detached and moved, or the tissue can remain attached as a **flap** and slid under the skin up to the chest. The tissue is sewn into place as a new breast. They cut you from hipbone to hipbone, what a frightening looking scar. The excess skin and fat that are removed from the lower abdomen can be considered a *"tummy tuck"*, which is a great benefit, there is a mesh placed into your abdomen to keep from bulging then they have to reconstruct your belly button. I couldn't believe that they could take your abdominal muscles and bring them up to your breast and transfer the fat from your abdomen to make breasts out of your own tissue. WOW! How great would that be! It would feel more like your own body! That sounded so much better then having fake jelly feeling foreign objects in my body.

I thought about the two options and I ended up going with the tram; I was very hesitant because my mind was set on the implant surgery, but the plastic surgeon said that my skin on the affected side would not stretch enough to hold implants since I had just finished radiation to that breast. It was too soon.

That is the reason I went with the tram flap, BIG MISTAKE. In the back of my mind, I kept hearing Cindy telling me not to do it, "do not let them talk you into the tram flap," but they did.

"I should have listened to Cindy!"

We arranged for doctors, (the breast surgeon and the plastic surgeon) to both be in the operating room together. These two doctors were the best and both were highly recommended. I had never felt more comfortable. My surgery was scheduled for July 12, 2004. The doctors told me that the total time of this surgery would be approximately nine hours; I had never been under anesthesia for that long, so needless to say I was horrified, plus I would have to spend four to six days in the hospital. That was hard for me because my son was three and really had never been away from me for that long. He still is too young to completely understand how sick I actually was. At that age they don't realize the depth of what is really happening. I had to make special arrangements for him during the day, I was going to have a lot of restrictions and one of them of course was no lifting, climbing, pushing, etc. My recovery would be about eight to twelve weeks; possibly longer because it was both breasts. I would have four tubes hanging out of my body two at the tram flap area and one at each of my breast.

Chapter Sixteen

"Menopause Time"

It was May 7 2004; time for one of the two most invasive surgeries the hysterectomy. I was really scared I just wanted all of this to be over. I was sick and tired of doctors by this time. I was scheduled to stay at the hospital for about three to four days. It was the first time since Owen was born that I had been away from him for that long of a time. I felt bad because in the past year every time I dropped him off to my mother in law, a friend, or a family member, I went to either a doctors appointment, or in for surgery. He started to pick up on that. He might have only been three but he knew. He is a very smart little boy. He would cry when I would leave him and that broke my heart, I told him that I loved him and mommy would see him later. "I felt so bad lying to him." He thinks I am coming home, but I am not.

I went in on a Friday at 7:00 am for a surgery, start time of 9:00am, Gary my mom and my good friend Evelyn were all there for me. This was the first time Sandy was unable to be with us. We sat in the pre op holding area waiting to go in. We were all laughing, joking, and talking about old times trying to take away some of the fear. Of course there was an emergency and I did not go in for surgery until 1:00pm. I was starving and so was everyone else; I had to fast the night before, so I told everyone else to go and get some food, but they wouldn't leave my side, afraid if they did the doctors would have taken me in before they could get back. I was getting very frustrated just sitting there waiting, everyone was getting impatient the surgery was about three hours which meant by the time it was over it would be about 4:00pm. Gary had already arranged to go to a Mets game with his friend Mark. I didn't have the heart to tell him he could not go. He needed to spend some time with his friends; he also was under a lot of stress, because I wasn't the only one going through this devastating disease. He had already had the tickets before I had my surgery scheduled. I remember asking the doctor and the nurse to make sure he was able to see me since my surgery was delayed. I knew Dr. P., would make special arrangements, for him. Once I was brought into the recovery room, the doctor brought Gary back to see me, so he knew I was okay. He held my hand and said he loved me and told me everything went great. The doctor didn't seem to think there was any cancer on the ovaries. "I was clean," but he would still send the ovaries out to pathology as a precaution.

I remember telling Gary that I loved him too and to give Owen a hug from me. I wanted him to go an enjoy himself and not worry about me. There was no need for him to sit there and watch me sleep and be in pain. My mom stayed with me the whole time until about 9:00pm that night. I remember being in so much pain. I was throwing up; it was horrible, throwing up with staples in your lower abdomen, it felt like the staples were popping out. My mom was holding my hand and I asked her to go check on my friend; who actually came into the hospital to have her baby while I was waiting to go into surgery. We were all watching her and her husband trying to find a parking spot in the maternity section. You could see that they both were so nervous they had no idea that we could see them. My mom went and checked on her and came back to tell me she had the baby and they both were fine. I told my mom to go home and get some rest.

The next morning I was thirsty, hungry and miserable, I could not wait for them to take the catheter out. The pain was so bad, every time I moved it hurt. I remember thinking if this hurts what is the mastectomy going to feel like!

I started feeling lonely and depressed I missed Gary and Owen and just could not wait to go home, but I knew that would not be for a few days. After having that catheter in for so long when it came out I felt like I had to go the bathroom all the time. I rang for the nurse so she could help me up to go to the bathroom. One of the nurses in training (a man) came in and tried to give me a bedpan. I sent him right back out that door and asked him to get someone who could bring me to the bathroom. He said that the nurse was busy and I had no choice but to go in the bedpan. I told him if he did not get someone to help I was getting up myself, well sure enough one of the nurses came in to help me and said it is very unusual for a patient who has had this type of surgery to get up so fast. I told her that I was not your typical patient. I was up moving around the day after surgery not even 24 hours later. The doctors and nurses on the floor were very impressed.

My mom and dad came to see me that next day and they sat with me for hours. When my brother arrived my mom and dad left, David stayed with me for a while, I knew he wasn't dealing with this to well, he wasn't him self. He hung out with me and we laughed and talked, when Gary came into the room, he and my brother talked a little while, my brother told me he was going home, if I needed anything to call.

I was so happy to see Gary, I missed him so much. He looked exhausted, he had been at the hospital all day Friday, and then left for the Mets game Friday night; he didn't get home until after midnight Friday. Owen had spent the night at my brother's house; we figured he would be distracted by my niece and nephew. I asked Gary why he didn't bring Owen, he said Owen was having fun with the kids, and he wasn't sure what kind of shape I was going to be in. He wanted to see me first he didn't want Owen to be scared. He told me that he would bring him back that evening if I felt up to it.

I could see how tired he was so I told him to go home and get some rest I would call him later. Once Gary left I fell asleep for a while, had my lunch and took a walk.

The nurses liked to see me up and moving around.

A few of my friends that I used to work with came to see me. I was excited to see them they were making me laugh; but it hurt too much. Sandy also stopped in to see me that afternoon; she hadn't seen me since before the surgery. She had a class to attend at the hospital, she couldn't miss. They all did not stay long, they could see I was very tired and in pain.

That evening, after I had dinner Gary brought Owen to see me. That just made all the pain go away. I knew he was frightened, he was afraid to touch me, not sure if he would hurt me. I let him sit with me on the bed, he kept hugging me and asking me when I was coming home, he missed me. When the doctor came in he said how happy he was that I was moving around, eating and going to the bathroom with no problems. I was making a remarkable recovery; most women do not get out of bed until 48 hrs after surgery. He told me that if tomorrow, which would be Sunday if I was feeling better I might be able to go home, as long as I promised to stay on one floor, no lifting, and in bed. The next day was Mothers' Day so I was happy to possibly be going home.

Sunday morning came and the doctor was in bright and early, he gave me the okay to go home. I called Gary to tell him the good news, I could go home. He was thrilled; he told me he would be there within the next hour. After I ate my breakfast and went to the bathroom the nurse helped me take a shower and get dressed. I then took a walk through the halls, since the nurses wanted me moving around as much as possible as this would help break down some of the anesthesia and also stretch my tight muscles.

I went back to my bed to rest, because I was getting tired, I heard a little voice calling "Mommy where are you, Mommy"! I knew it was Owen; he came around the corner with flowers and a present for me for Mothers' Day, and said, "Can you come home? I miss you". He sat in bed with me for a while, Gary and my mother in law went for a walk. The doctor came in and said everything looked good, and I could go home, and then said "this is an early Mothers Day Present," so take it easy. After the nurse came in to discharge me and gave me instructions on how to care for myself and when to take my medicine off we went, home at last. It is always nice to go home to your own bed, food, and bathroom. I had so much help at home, when Gary left for work in the mornings he always made sure someone was with me at all times. Friends and family were cooking and cleaning for me, helping with Owen. I had to have my friends come over and bathe me, change my dressing from the surgery, and even dress me. I am so lucky to have so many people around who love me.

As the weeks went by I started to feel better. I was up and driving after about two weeks. I just couldn't sit in the house anymore. I still was unable to pick up Owen, even through he was three and a half he still needed help with getting in and out of the car seat. When Dr. P., told me that menopause would start immediately he was right, I was having hot flashes, my ears would get really hot and then I would get cold. Night sweats were the worst. I would actually wake up in the middle of the night and be soaked like I just got out of a pool. The mood swings were bad; I tried not to complain too much because by this time everyone had to be tired of listening to me. I started to compare everything to the chemotherapy and there is nothing worse then that. I will take menopause any day. My friend Laura, who I worked with, had been diagnosed six months before me with breast cancer. Laura was the only one who could understand how I was feeling.

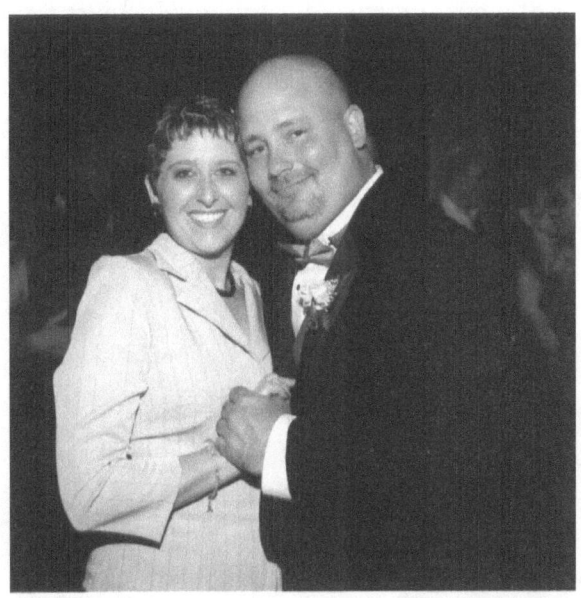

Karen and Gary at Pam and Franks wedding

Two weeks after my hysterectomy Gary's brother was getting married. Gary was his best man and I was supposed to be helping Pamela (the bride to be) get everything ready at the reception hall the night before her "big day". But my doctor instructed me not to do any lifting, and to take it easy not to tire myself out. It was very hard for me to just sit still and watch. Pam and I decided to gather some friends and family to meet us at the reception hall to help with the set up. We were very pleased with the hall it looked beautiful.

The morning of the wedding Pam called me to ask if I could come over to her parents house because she wasn't feeling so well. She was nervous and felt really sick to her stomach. I went to the deli and picked her up some ginger ale, crackers, and a bagel. After about two hours she called to say she felt alot better.

Gary and I had a house full of family from out of town staying with us for the weekend. I was doing exactly what the doctors didn't want me to do. I was running around like crazy. The guys needed help getting dressed and I had to make sure my company was entertained. During the wedding the photographer and I were talking and he couldn't believe that I had just under went a complete hysterectomy two weeks earlier. I was having alot of pain, and tried not to show it, I just wanted everyone to focus on Pam and Frank, it was their day, I didn't need anyone to be worried about me.

The wedding was beautiful and we all had a fantastic time, and of course Pamela looked stunning, absolutley beautiful.

When we arrived home that evening I was completely exhausted, I went right to bed. The next morning I knew I over did myself and made sure that I stayed in bed for the rest of the day.

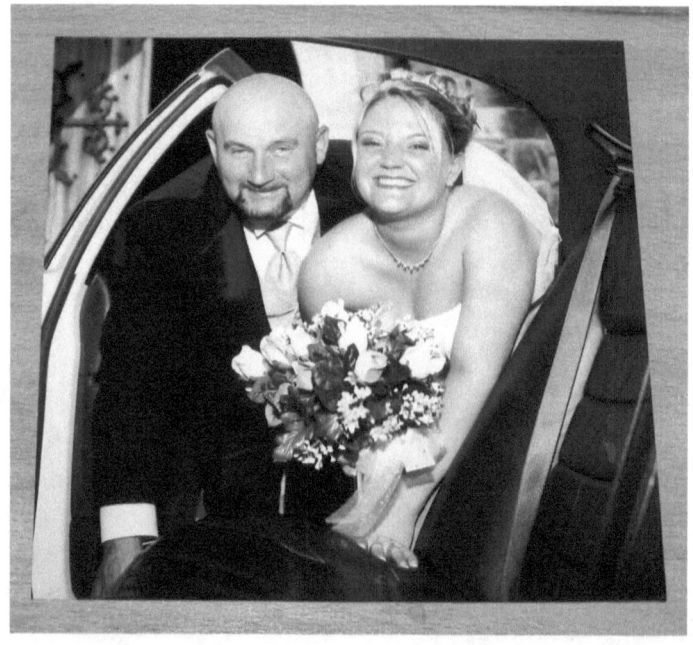

Pam and Frank May 22, 2004.

Chapter Seventeen

Summer Has Begun!

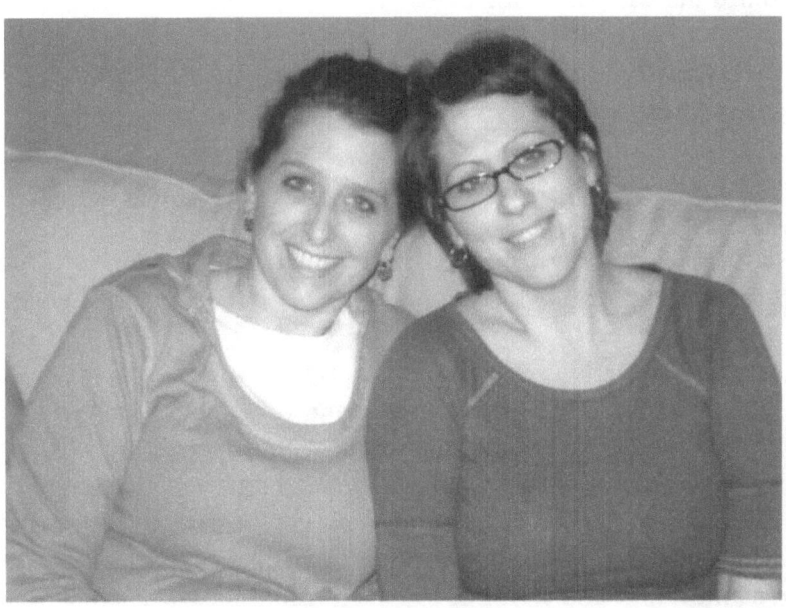

True Friends
Karen and Kim

It was July 2004, Sandy had a surprise birthday party planned for her husband Dave and everyone was going to be there. It was outside at her house, she invited about 50-60 people, I knew almost everyone. It was nice to see people I hadn't been able to talk too in a long while. People are so nice to you when they know that you have had cancer, every one looked at me differently.

(I would hear all the time what an inspiration I was to a lot of people, how positive I was.) It started to get frustrating, hearing how positive I was.

During the party I was introduced to one of Sandy's friends, Kim. I knew who she was because I would see her at the ball field, her son and my nephew both played baseball together, but I never was ever properly introduced. I knew from the moment we spoke that we would become great friends. She is very caring, sincere, loving, strong minded, and has a great personality; she is beautiful and has a great spirit about her. Kim is the kind of friend who will always be there no matter what is happening in your life, good or bad. She has two children a boy and a little girl her and her family were leaving for vacation the day after the party. She offered to come over and help me when I got home from the hospital after my mastectomy and reconstruction surgery, she also is a RN and knew exactly what to do to help me. Of course I welcomed her with open arms.

"You know a true friend when one comes along, and she is definitely that true friend."

Today is the Day

I was ready to have my bilateral mastectomy with immediate reconstruction. I was scared and anxious to see how big my boobs were actually going to be.

It was July 12th, and I had to be at the hospital at 7:00am in the morning. Gary, Sandy, Dave and my mother all came with me for this one; Owen was with my mother in law and then went with my Dad, until Gary came home. The surgery would be about nine to ten hours and an eight to twelve week recovery period. The nurse came out to get me from the waiting room, she brought me into pre op room that looked like a 4 star hotel room, it was so comfortable, and warm. It had a television, nice bed, and a beautiful bathroom. The nurse gave me a beautiful terry cloth bath robe to put on, I felt like someone important. "I did not feel like I was in a hospital."

The doctor came in to draw all over my body with a marker to determine were they would be cutting, moving, and removing parts. When he was finished I looked like a science project on a black board for everyone to copy. When the doctor was finished, he sent my family and friends into my room before the nurses took me off to the operating room. This surgery made me so nervous; I had never been under anesthesia for that long of a time. I was afraid I would not wake up and never see Owen or my family again.

You would think that after having so many surgeries you would eventually get used to it and know that you will wake up.

The first thing they did was removed my original breasts saving my skin. Then they cut me from one side of my hipbone to the other. This was so they could tunnel the abdominal muscles up to my breasts and then take the fat I had in my abdomen to make new breasts. Once they finished that, they then gave me a tummy tuck, because they had to pull some of the skin from my abdomen down and make it flat, to do this they had to place a mesh patch in my abdomen and reconstruct my belly button, which never healed properly.

When I woke up, I heard all of this commotion going on around me. I could not open my eyes for some reason but I heard the nurses. The plastic surgeon kept saying he was not leaving until I was stable. Then I heard Sandy's voice, I had (tachy cardia) they needed to give me more fluids and lower my heart rate, this was because I was under anesthesia for so long without fluids. I must have fallen back to sleep because when I woke up everyone was looking at me and talking to me. I was so high on drugs that I could not feel a thing and I immediately looked down my hospital gown and said "WOW I have boobs!" Everyone was laughing.

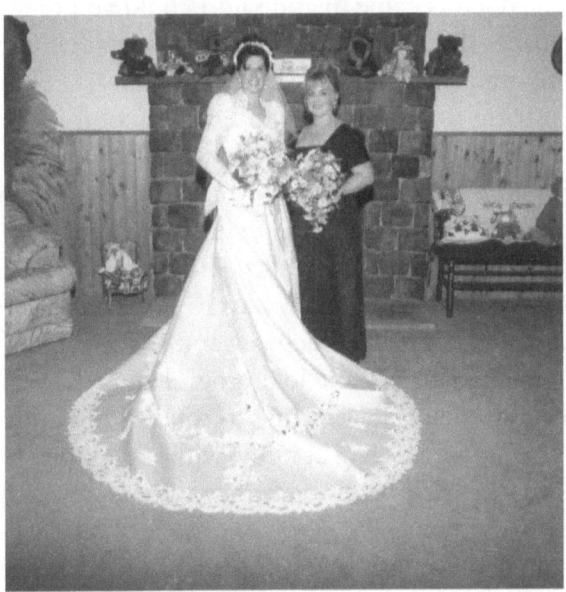

Best friends
Karen and Dawn

At about 6:30pm I told everyone to go home, they had been with me all day, my best friend Dawn just got there to relieve them so they could go. She was going to sit with me for a while so I was not by myself. Gary, my mom, Sandy and Dave said good bye and they would see me tomorrow. I told them to be careful driving home and that I loved all of them. "Give Owen a big kiss for me".

I joked around with Dawn for a while; do not ask me what I said because I do not even remember. I knew she was tired because she came from work. It was now 9:30 pm, and she still had to drive another hour home. I told her I would be fine, so she left. The next day was totally different, I was in so much pain, and oh my God did it hurt! Not only was my chest sore, but my abdomen looked as if it were ripped apart. I had the tubes they told me about; the tubes had all kinds of blood and fat liquid in them it was gross. Every four hours they had to be emptied and measured.

My mom, dad, Gary and Owen came to see me the next day, but they didn't really stay too long. I think Owen was a little scared. He again was too young to really understand what was happening all he knew was that mommy was sick and had to get new boobs. I told Gary that they could leave, I wouldn't be upset. I spoke to Gary three times a day, I told him not to come to the hospital everyday because he had to take care of Owen and work. I few days later, the doctors came in and said I could go home. I had to keep track of the (grenades that's what I called them); tubes that were hanging out of me, two at my tram flap site and one at each breast. They were so long that I had to pin them to my bathrobe so I would not trip over them. It was so disgusting. I had to empty them myself when no one was able to come around. Gary couldn't even look at them; you could see the bloody fatty fluid moving from the long clear tube to the drain at the end.

Kim was still on vacation and called me when I got home from the hospital. She wanted to make sure I was okay. She said she would be home in two days and would come by to help as soon as she could. Sandy stopped in everyday to help me out. I would joke around and tell everyone that I felt like a cow with udders, and it was time to squeeze the milk out, except it was not milk. After about six days at home with these tubes the doctor took them out Thank God! I felt better once they were removed, but I had a lot of healing to do.

A few days after the tubes were removed I called Kim because when I bent over in the shower my boob squirted out all kinds of bloody fluid. I freaked out, "what in the world is this." Every time I moved the bloody fluid poured out of my breast. It wouldn't stop; I didn't know what to do. I called the plastic surgeon and he told me to come in right away. So Kim drove me to the office, we sat there for over an hour in the room waiting. When Kim stuck her head out of the room the nurse said, "Sorry I forgot you were in there." When the doctor finally came in he looked at my right breast and said it was nothing to worry about. The bloody fluid is left over fluid that had not absorbed into my tissue. The breast looks fine, this should not happen again. I was definitely having trouble dealing with the out come of this surgery, I was not happy with it at all.

"What did I do to myself?"

After several more surgeries following the *"big one"* I needed some corrections to both breasts, the doctors had to make me new nipples and areolas. Mine had to be removed during the reconstruction surgery. This surgery was less invasive. I was only under anesthesia for about one and half hours and a bonus for me some liposuction on my hips to fill in where my new breast tissue did not settle properly. I was happy that my hips would be small again, since I did gain thirty pounds from all of the chemo and steroids I had to take. Once the nipples healed about one month later, they started the tattooing of the areolas. How cool this was, I was stunned that the plastic surgeon could tattoo my breasts, I even got to pick the color for the areolas. All of the reconstruction was finally finished in December 2004.

Chapter Eighteen

"Time Fly's"

Another year had passed we made it to 2005, and I was hoping to get the New Year off with getting myself back together. I still had a long road ahead, I was still recovering physically and mentally I had a lot of work to do. My surgeries were finally finished, my body was so scarred up and needed a lot of healing. The winter was always the hardest on me because of the cold weather. My body would ache all the time I felt like a little old lady and I was only thirty five years old.

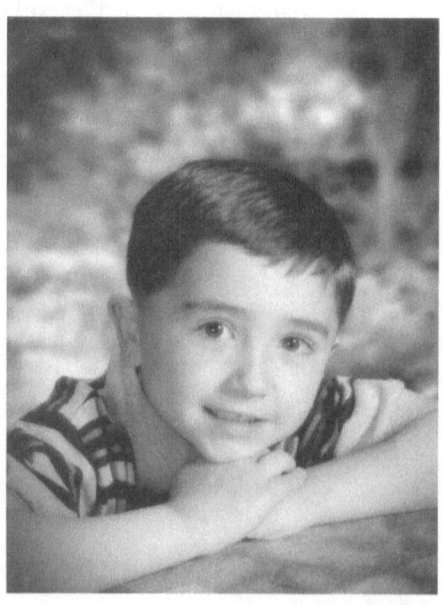

My son Owen Maneri

Owen was starting kindergarten in September and I was looking forward to him being in school for almost a full day. He definitely needed to be with his friends. Owen is the type of kid who needs structure in his life. There were so many ups and downs in his life through out the past two years, socially and emotionally, this would be good for him. He is attending pre-k at the same school he is going to be attending kindergarten, so he was definitely familiar with the school. I was nervous with him because he is so sensitive and shy. He isn't very out going, but does make friends easily. Some of his friends from pre-k would be with him in kindergarten. He definitely has some separation anxiety from me.

"Fun in the Sun"

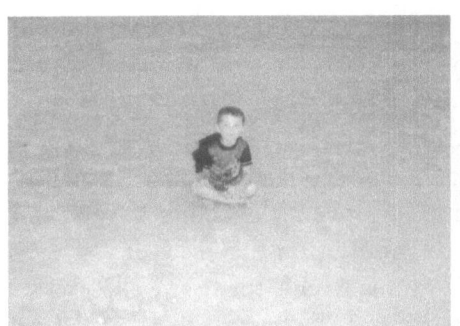 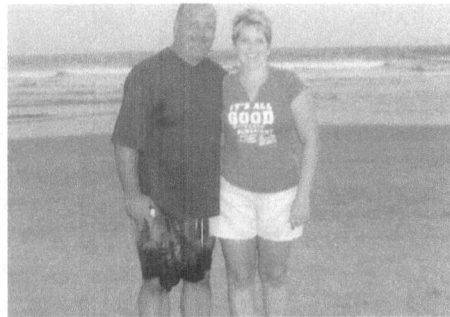

North Myrtle Beach
Owen on the beach, Gary and Karen

Winter and spring flew by and summer was right around the corner. Gary and I had summer vacation plans this year. We never went on vacation. I was looking forward to getting out of the house. I did become a bit of a hermit. I was embarrassed about the way my body looked. Our vacation was planned for the end of July. We were going to the beach with our friends for ten days. Gary is not really a big beach person but we needed a vacation and what better way to go then with a group of friends and their kids. We packed up everyone July 21, and drove off to North Myrtle Beach for 10 days. Sandy, Daniel, Owen and I rode in Sandy's car. She had a SUV with a DVD player. This would keep the kids occupied. Gary, Dave, Davey and his friend rode in my car, and Mark, Elaine, and their kids were in their car. This was going to be a challenge because I never wanted to leave my house, and I had to put on a bathing suit. I was very insecure. When we finally arrived, after a long fourteen hour drive, we pulled up to the house where we all were staying. It was gorgeous; it had four bedrooms and two bathrooms. Walking out of the kitchen onto the back porch we were looking right at the ocean. There was also a pool at the house. The kids just had a blast. It was so nice to be away from home where all of the bad things had been happening. I really felt as if this was what I needed.

The days were hot and the nights were cool, it definitely was very therapeutic for me just listening to the ocean. Walking through the sand was very calming to me. Gary and I were able to spend some alone time one the beach at night time when Owen was sleeping. It was very romantic to walk hand and hand up and down the beach. I felt alive again, and I hadn't felt like that for years. I thought that I would be a little more insecure about the way my body looked in summer clothes and a bathing suit, you definitely could see the awful scars I had. It was not as bad as I thought because I did not know anyone and didn't care if people stared at me, because I would never see them again.

It was a long, hot ten days, especially since Gary and I weren't really beach people. Gary, Owen and I spent the days going to the aquarium and playing miniature golf and we went shopping. We really couldn't spend too much time outside unless we were in the pool or on the beach it was over 100 degrees every day and very humid. I didn't handle the heat well, my feet and hands would swell so much that they hurt. The doctors had warned me that this might be a side effect from all the chemo. I really enjoyed watching Owen playing on the beach in the sand and in the ocean with the other kids and little Daniel; he was having so much fun. It was great to see him with a smile on his face. Gary was able to relax and spend time with Mark and Dave, and I was able to spend quality time with Elaine and Sandy. It was just an all around great time. By the end of the week I was ready to go home, and be back in my comfort zone. That is what happens when you have lost so much of yourself, you tend to stay close to what is comfortable for you.

"I Felt So Alone"

I tried to hide myself from everyone, because every time I saw or spoke to someone and they asked me how I was feeling, I felt like they were looking at my boobs. "People hear breast cancer and they automatically start to wonder about the boobs." I thought by now the scars would have looked a little better, but they didn't, I became more depressed and had a lot of anxiety, I was tired of being positive all the time. Everyone was always telling me what an inspiration I was and how positive I was all the time, so I felt like I had to keep that reputation of myself. If they only knew how I felt inside. I was dying inside, I did not know who I was anymore, and I had no ambition to lose weight. Every time I had to go for a test something showed on a report and I had to have more biopsies or additional tests to rule things out. I felt like a ticking time bomb. Every day I think to myself, is today the day my cancer comes back. I have to live with this feeling everyday, and unless you have had cancer then you will never know what that feels like.

Through out the next few months my body was trying to heal and the routine test were always coming up, which meant the dreadful feeling of "has the cancer returned? I knew that if it did return than I had to deal with it and do whatever it took to fight the disease. In some aspects, it may be easier because I would know what I would be up against, but in others, I have a son who would understand more because he has grown. It also would be very discouraging to be diagnosed for the second time.

Work Out Time

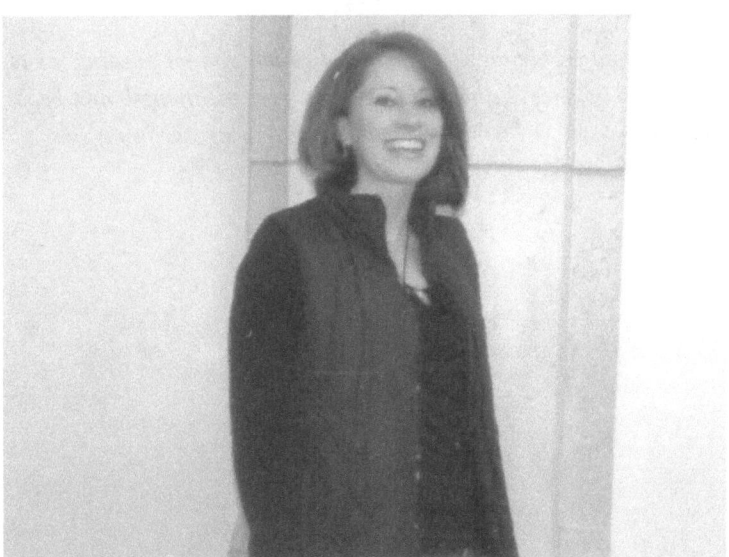

Aimee my friend and personal Trainer

With a lot of therapy I felt like I was making some progress with my insecurities, I finally decided to get off my butt and start to work out. So I hired a personal trainer, her name is Aimee. I met Aimee many years ago, we took gymnastics class together. I was in seeing Dr. P., and had asked him if he knew of a personal trainer that could whip me into shape again. He suggested Aimee; she was actually in the office the same time I was. After my appointment Dr. P., asked me to wait in the waiting room and he would bring her out to talk to me. Well, when we looked at each other, we were so surprised. I hadn't seen her in years. It was meant to be. Someone was telling me it's time to exercise. I went to see her every Tuesday morning. She measured and weighed me, and we started a workout plan. I set goals for myself and made sure that I followed them everyday. I needed to do this. Once I started to work out, I started to feel so much better physically and mentally. I couldn't believe how good I felt about myself again, I watched the weight fall right off my body. During the next six months I lost thirty pounds and twenty inches I was amazed. I was so proud of myself. I also made myself a promise and that promise was to never allow myself to feel bad about my body again. Working out with Aimee every week for seven months was life changing. I watched myself transform into a different person inside and out. I noticed my mood swings were better and my outlook on life was different; I was happy again. For that:

> "I thank you Aimee for all of your dedication and for pushing me to make me feel complete again. Aimee you gave me strength and hope, something I lost along the way." You are a shining star in my life.

Chapter Nineteen

Tattoo of Hope

My tattoo

One afternoon my husband and I were goofing around and he had mentioned in a kidding way that I should get a tattoo on my lower back. I thought he was crazy a tattoo, I had my share with needles going through chemotherapy; I am not getting a tattoo. He thought that it would look really sexy. I never in my wildest dreams would have expected that to come out of Gary's month. He doesn't have any tattoos, he is such a simple laid back person I didn't think he was serious. That idea stayed with me for a while and the more I thought about it the more I liked it. If I was going to do it, it was going to be something meaningful and symbolic of me. I had the artist at the tattoo parlor draw something up for me. I told him I was a breast cancer survivor, and I wanted some kind of pink ribbon with some colorful flowers. He told me that he would draw up some designs and to come back in a week and see if I liked what he drew. Of course I loved it! I made the appointment, I was so excited, and I can't believe I am going through with this. I knew it was going to hurt like hell, how could it not? A few of my friends who have tattoos told me that it wasn't really that bad. So when I went in for my tattoo Sandy and Kim came with me, even my sister in law Pam stopped by to see me, which made me happy. When the tattoo artist made that very first line I thought to myself, what did I do? Oh my God it hurt like hell!

Sandy stayed with me the whole time, (it took forever 4 hours of torture) I couldn't wait for it to be over. I was sweating like crazy, I turned white as a ghost and I thought I was going to pass out. I had Sandy call Gary so he wouldn't be surprised as to how big the tattoo was. I wasn't sure if he realized it wasn't just going to be this small little ribbon with flowers.

Finally he was finished, it may have hurt badly, but I did it. It is beautiful, I love it and I am so glad I went through with it! Breast cancer is such a big part of my life and always will be so why not have it drawn on my body. Gary was surprised when he saw the size, but he really likes it. My son was so excited; he thought that the tattoo artist drew it with permanent magic markers. He couldn't wait to tell everyone!

I'm A New Woman!

When I went in for my last surgery in March of 2007, I went in with this great feeling of accomplishment knowing finally that I would look better then I had in a long time. The weight was gone, my hair was back longer and better then before, and I would look like a woman again. I was four years cancer free. I was going in to have implants because when I lost the weight I had gained from all the medicine I was on; I lost it in my new boobs. So once again, I needed to make some changes. I went to the same doctor who preformed the original reconstruction, since we had a long history together and I was very comfortable with him. I went into see him and he looked over my breasts and agreed that he could and would make them look better. I told him that if I'm going to do this then I want them to look bigger and not one size smaller. "If I'm going to do it then lets do it right!" I went with saline implants. I could have had the silicone implants but I didn't want to take that risk of something happening to them and developing infection.

I scheduled my surgery date for mid March 2007. I walked out of the office feeling more secure then I had felt in years. I went home and told my husband that the doctor agreed to do the surgery and it would be covered under my insurance, because I was a breast cancer survivor. He was happy that I was happy and this would hopefully put an end to a long horrific battle against breast cancer. I was hoping that I would be able to close this chapter of my life. This would be a same day surgery, which was great because it required no hospital stay.

"Terrified"

I arrived with my mom and Sandy about 10:00am at the hospital. I could not wait to go in and have this finished and see my new breasts. These would be what I have been waiting for, for a long time.

I went in to the beautiful pre op room I was in when I had the first surgery in 2004. The doctor came in to go over a few last minute touch ups, and make sure we both were on the same page. Once he left, the nurse came in to start all the paper work. Then in came the anesthesiologist, he asked many questions, and explained what was going to happen. I had so many surgeries that I knew what the routine was and what to expect. However, he had to go over everything with me anyway this was routine. The doctors told my mom and Sandy that the surgery would take about three hours.

The nurse walked me into the operating room and put me on the table. The doctor held my hand and told me that he was so proud of me, and that I was a gift sent here from God to help other women. He said "I inspired him."

The anesthesiologist started my IV and injected some medicine into my veins, I started to cry and the surgeon asked me why I was upset, I told him I was happy but also scared. He told me not to worry; he would take good care of me. Under I went, fast asleep, I had general anesthesia, [which meant they had to insert a tube down my throat that breathes for you.] During the surgery something went wrong!

Suddenly I started hearing noises, beeping noises, and then people talking. I thought at first I was in the recovery room, but then I started feeling this horrific pain, I felt like my body was on fire. I started to scream and call to the doctors but no one was answering me. I tried to move my legs and arms—nothing. I could not believe no one could hear me. I started screaming even louder, "so I thought." I then heard the nurse and the doctor talking over my left shoulder and I felt this pain like my breast was going to explode into a million pieces. I realized they could not hear me; they had no idea that I was awake. "How do they not know I'm awake," I kept saying to myself "please God let them be finished." Then the pain came back and I just wanted to die. I can't believe they are not finished, how much longer, please someone help me!

I panicked when I tried to open my eyes and I could not see anything. I could feel myself breathing though my nose, not my mouth. I could still feel the tube down my throat. This was a nightmare; I was being tortured on the operating table. How does something like this actually happen? Then everything went black!!!

Next thing I knew, I woke up in the recovery room. I knew this time I was in recovery because I could see the nurse. When she realized I was alert she asked me what kind of pain I was in, but before I could tell her what happened during my surgery, she shot me up with Demerol which is pain medicine and out I went again.

About half an hour went by then the nurse gave me more Demerol and put me in a wheelchair, wheeled me to where Sandy and my mom where waiting. When I arrived back to my room they asked how everything went, my mother said the doctor said the boobs looked great. I couldn't react to what they were saying, the only thing that came out of my mouth was "I heard and felt the surgery."

Dead silence in the room, Sandy said "WHAT?" I repeated myself; the nurse looked at Sandy and my mom then shut the door.

Two minutes later the surgeon who did the surgery came in to see me. The nurse must have told him what I said, because he asked me; 'Karen what did you hear' "I told him, and he said you heard correctly;" he apologized and kept repeating himself, saying "you must have been terrified?" "I am so sorry that this has happened to you." Then he closed the door and walked away. I had experienced anesthesia awareness. I was awake and terrified!

I was so sick from the anesthesia and the shock that I started throwing up; also, I was on so much pain medicine that I could not even function like a normal person. Sandy and my mother tried to give me some crackers and ginger ale. The nurse asked my mom to help me get dressed and she gave us, (well them,) my discharge papers. Nothing else was said about what happened in the operating room. Out the door I went, on the way home I was so sick, I was sitting in the front seat of my mother's car and Sandy was sitting in the back, my mom was driving. Sandy was talking to our friend Kim and telling her what had happened to me, (waking up on the operating table,) Kim could not believe this had happened. It was unacceptable this should have never happened. Sandy also called Gary to let him know what kind of shape

I was in. I didn't want to scare Owen. We wanted to prepare Gary for what state of mind I was in, it wasn't good. When we got home my husband was pissed off that this happened to me, after everything that I had been through to have this happen was completely uncalled for. At this moment there was nothing we could do until all of the medicine wore off.

About one week went by and I stopped taking the pain pills. I started having problems sleeping having nightmares. I could not lay flat; every time I closed my eyes I relived this terrible horrific experience. I felt as if I were being tortured all over again. It was the worst experience of my life. I became more depressed, my anxiety was really bad, I was afraid to close my eyes, and I kept hearing everything play over and over in my head. I went in to make myself feel better about the way I looked and I came out a very different person.

I now suffer from Post-Traumatic Stress Disorder; I take all different kinds of pills, especially at night to help me sleep. My primary care physician wants to see me every three months to make sure I am okay. I sure hope I don't have to have any more surgery. These new boobs better hold up nice, because I don't think mentally I can handle having to go under anesthesia again.

Chapter Twenty

"Beyond Reflection"

The past five years has been a constant battle, not only for me but also for my son, husband and whole family. When diagnosed with a disease especially cancer, your whole world changes in an instant, sometimes for the better and other times for the worst.

Being a breast cancer survivor, I have learned so much from so many different people. When you have lived with and survived an unpredictable frightening disease, in the end you are not the same person you where before your diagnoses. I found that living for today is the only way to live. "I will live, love and laugh every day." I can not worry about tomorrow, the next day, or the next six months. I am focused on my life with my husband and son. They come first, everything else comes second. I have washed my hands of all negative energy surrounding me and my family. I have become a more positive person then I ever was before breast cancer. I have found strength within myself. I believe this journey has taken me to a better place in my life. Part of me is thankful for the disease, because it made me into the person I always knew I could be.

I hope that every person who is either living with breast cancer, or any other type of cancer takes into consideration all the help that is out there for you and your family. There are support groups for everyone involved. So many people will have their own ideas about what you should do and what type of treatment to take, but remember you have a choice and you make that decision, no one else does. Do not ever let the influence of someone else make choices for you. I am proof that with having a strong positive attitude and being open minded with treatment plans saved my life. You need to stand up for yourself and be forceful about your health, take charge, get a copy of every test result, be on top of your insurance carrier, don't let anyone tell you "No you can't have something done."

"Losing Your Self Image"

I am writing today to hopefully help other people who are young survivors battling this disease or just a friend or loved one trying to find some answers. You do not have to lose your inner strength, courage or fight when you lose part of yourself. As a woman you must be strong and know that you can beat this disease. Do not let it get you. You become someone you may have never thought you could be. Reach out and ask for help or give help back to people who are going through what you have already experienced. Don't be afraid to say you're scared or show how you feel. When I had my hysterectomy and bilateral mastectomy with reconstruction, I did not feel like a woman anymore. A lot of people do not understand what it means to walk around without your womanly organs, your own breasts that have been taken from you, your self-image. I walked around for the longest time saying who am I, I know I am a mom, wife, daughter, aunt, sister and friend, but for myself I felt like I didn't have an identity anymore. You do overcome this and it takes a lot of soul searching, time and therapy.

If you are a woman who has beat this life threatening disease, or you are a woman or man fighting to survive, please be strong, and stay positive. It can be done, have faith in yourself.

If you are a loved one who has lost someone to breast cancer then please help support. There are so many organizations for breast cancer around that need your donations. It is very hard to understand what it feels like to be that person with cancer, unless you have experienced it yourself you can not image how we feel.

To be a woman and have to lose your hair, breast, or any other part of your body is devastating. Sometimes people who are trying to support you do not comprehend how it feels, often it is easy to say it is just hair, it will grow back, no, it is not just hair, I know it will grow back. We are not being selfish or difficult, we do know what the consequences are when it comes to treatment plans, we know that cancer kills, but please understand what we are feeling how overwhelming it all is.

If your friends can't support you because they feel your not doing the right thing then please don't allow them to be part of your support system.

If you want something done you have to push for it, you are in control, so take control of yourself starting with self breast exams, routine mammograms, ultra sounds, and if you have a family history then please keep up on all of your yearly physicals. You must be your own advocate when it comes to your health, by doing this you may just save your life. I did! If had not felt the lump that Friday evening, and acted on it, I would not be writing this today.

When I tested positive for the Brca 1 gene mutation I new that I would have to live will this for the rest of my life. This would be a permanent spot in the back of my mind at all times. With one little sniffle, backache, headache, lump, bruise, you name it, I will wonder is it back. This means at any time in my life this deadly disease can strike me again. In the meantime I will live everyday as if it were my last. A lot of people take the smallest things for granted or go around every day mad at the world, whether for jealous reasons, or just unhappy in their own life. Well, don't let the time slip away hating the world. Enjoy every waking moment you have with yourself and your family and friends, because one day it will all be gone. You must always take time out for yourself and stop doing for everyone else. Because in the long run of things YOU are what matters.

I AM A SURVIVOR!!!

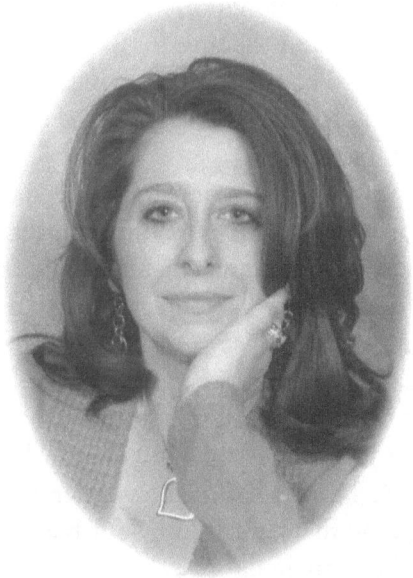

Karen Maneri 2008

I will be cancer free for 5 years May 20, 2008; looking back now I can see beyond the reflection in the mirror. I have survived this deadly disease, and hope to live a long happy life with my family and friends. I will grow old with the man of my dreams, watch my beautiful son grow from a boy to a man, and let God lead him in whatever direction he needs to go. I'm very blessed to have had the most incredible support system on my side. My life in the past five years has been a roller coaster ride and I've had to struggle with so many ups and downs, that nobody should ever have to endure, but life is full of surprises. God only deals out what he thinks you can handle, God has plans for all of us and I strongly believe God needs me to be around to help others. I have learned to live with the fact that I may get cancer again, but I won't sit back and wait for it to happen. I still have my bad days and I will always be reminded as to what I have been through. Every time I look at myself in the mirror I see a woman who has been through hell and back, scarred up like I have been cut in half and sewed back together. But I made it through those terrible times and I am alive.

Ten Year Wedding Anniversary

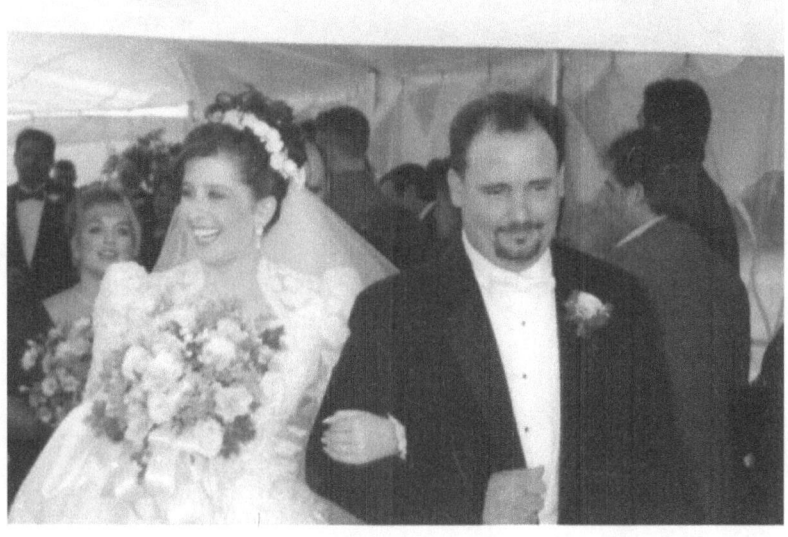

Gary and Karen
October 24, 1998

This October 2008, Gary and I will be celebrating our wedding anniversary. In ten years we have had our share of heartache and happiness, we have cried, laughed, and struggled. We have had to deal with a lot of illness, which puts amazing pressure on a marriage. A lot of relationships don't survive the strains of death and cancer in such a short period of time. Gary and I vowed to be together in sickness and in health; till death do us part: we are each others' support system and will love one another long after we journey beyond this life here on earth.

> *Gary, I Love you with all my heart, you are my world. Thank you for being so strong and standing by my side. The past five years have been the most difficult years of our marriage. We made it through cancer we can make it through anything.*

"We are true soul mates!"

"Miles of Hope"

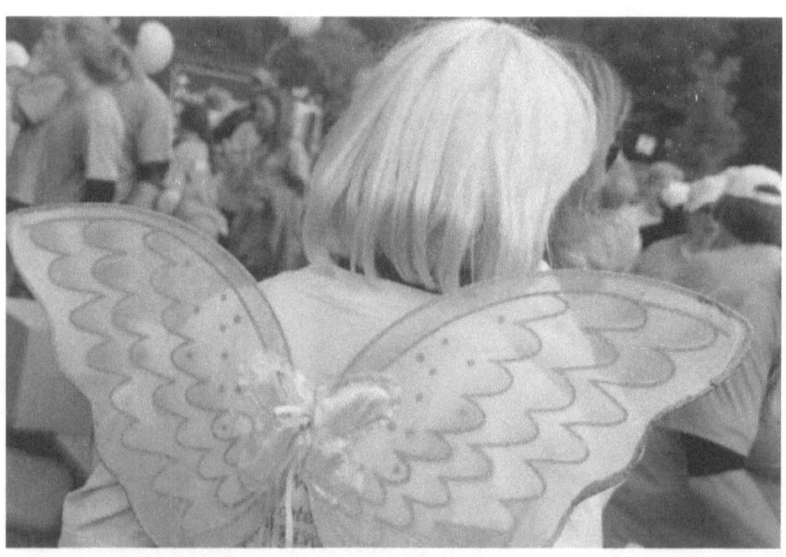

I am now 38 yrs old and I can finally say I'm starting to get part of my life back. I will never be the same person I was before breast cancer, but I know I'm a better person after breast cancer. I have found peace in my life with helping others and talking to young women who have all the questions I had when I was first diagnosed.

I help volunteer for a local breast cancer foundation called "Miles of Hope BCF of the Hudson Valley". I became involved in 2004 when my friend Laura who was also diagnosed with breast cancer, told me about the organization.

Miles of Hope BCF is an out reach for people affected by breast cancer in the Hudson Valley, New York. This includes (Columbia, Dutchess, Putnam,

Westchester, Rockland, Orange, Ulster and Greene counties), all proceeds donated go directly to the women and men of the Hudson Valley who have been stricken with breast cancer and need financial assistance. They are a non-profit organization and help pay for mortgages, cobra payments, physical therapy, car payment, utility bills etc., nothing goes to research.

For more information go to:

www.milesofhopebcf.org.

"Celebrating Life"

I will be hosting a dinner party for all my closest friends and family who stood by me and my family through this most difficult time in our lives, and asking them to come and celebrate life. I will not be accepting gifts, but I will be asking for everyone to make a small donation in honor of me to Miles of Hope BCF, of the Hudson Valley. I will be presenting the donations to the founders of this organization after my party.

This is mine and my husband's way of giving back to a fantastic group of women who have put so much time and effort into helping others

Help Fight Breast Cancer and Support!

You only do live once!

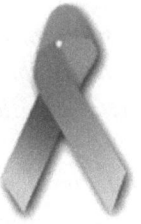

Acknowledgements

"Thank You for Saving My Life and Spirit"

I am thankful to all of the doctors, nurses and medical staff who have stood by my side from day one. Never once did anyone ever make me feel like they didn't care, you all will forever be in my heart.

Thank You to Dr. M., my medical oncologist and his staff, all the nurse's who stood by my side and made me smile every time I walked in the door for treatment. Cindy, a BIG thank you for being so honest and straight forward with me, you are the best I Love You.

Dr. P., thank you, for being you, because if you hadn't ordered the tests I may not be here today, you have a very special place in my heart.

To my breast surgeons and plastic surgeon, thank you for making me look like a woman again, you brought back my spirit I feel whole again. You all are remarkable surgeons with big hearts, God Bless.

Dr. G., my primary care physician, thank you for never giving up on me, and understanding all of my concerns, you never once let me down. You are a great doctor!

To Kristin; thank you for listening, and giving me the push to become myself again, and helping me through some of the most terrifying, challenging struggles that came my way in the past four years.

Owen my darling little angel, you have so much love in your heart. You are loving, caring, smart, thoughtful, and a talented little boy. Mommy is so proud of you I will love you always and forever, you are my life.

To my parents, I love both of you so much more then words can say. Thank you for all of your help and support along this long journey. I am very proud to be your daughter and lucky to have both of you in my life.

To my brother and his family, I love you all, thank you for being you and for loving me.

Sandy, I just want to say Thank You for everything that you did for me and my family while going through this difficult time. You are a true friend you will always have a special place in my heart. I Love You!

To all of my friends and family I love you all!! Thank you for being so supportive.

God Bless You All!!!!

www.ingramcontent.com/pod-product-compliance
Lightning Source LLC
Chambersburg PA
CBHW031259280526
45784CB00004B/1910